OSTEOPOROSIS COOKBOOK

The Ultimate Dietary Guide with 60 Delicious & Nutritious, Bone-Strengthening Recipes for Maintaining and Improving Your Bone Health

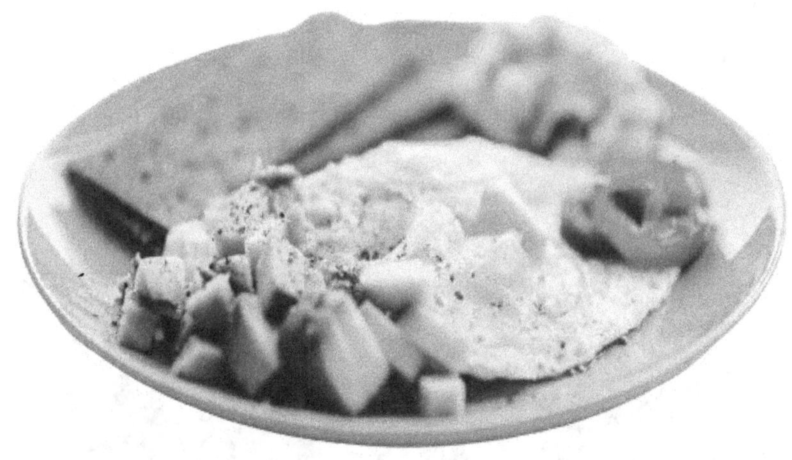

DR. COLE HULL

COPYRIGHT

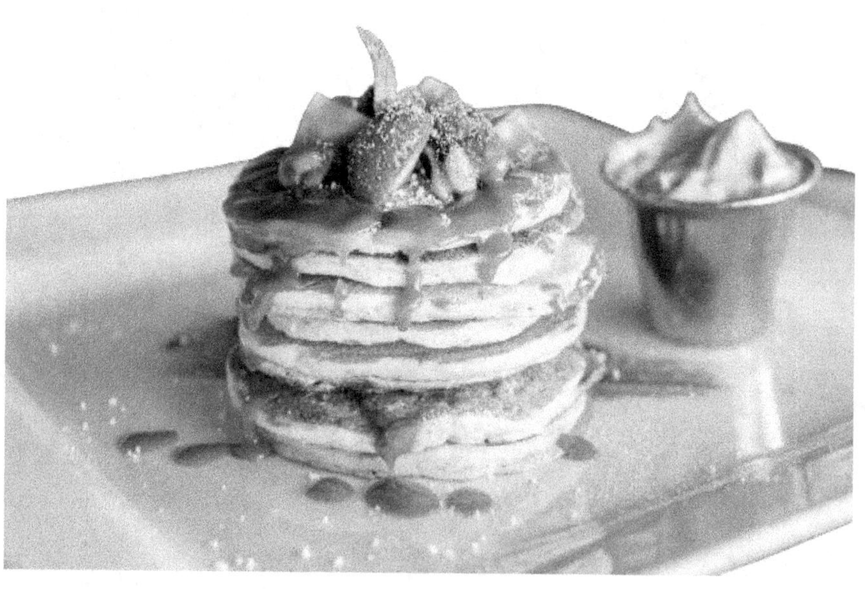

TABLE OF CONTENT

1. INTRODUCTION

UNDERSTANDING OSTEOPOROSIS: A BRIEF OVERVIEW

Osteoporosis is a bone condition characterized by a decrease in bone density and an increase in fragility, which can result in a greater likelihood of fractures. Bone loss can occur without any noticeable symptoms, earning it the nickname of a "silent disease." Many individuals are unaware of their osteoporosis condition until they experience a bone fracture. Recent studies indicate that osteoporosis is a widespread concern affecting a large number of individuals globally. Furthermore, its occurrence is on the rise due to the aging population.

Osteoporosis development is influenced by a variety of factors, including genetics, age, gender, and lifestyle choices. Postmenopausal women face a higher risk due to decreased estrogen levels. However, men can also experience significant impacts, especially as they age. It is essential to implement early prevention and intervention strategies to effectively manage this condition.

Understanding the importance of nutrition is crucial when it comes to preventing and managing osteoporosis. Ensuring strong and healthy bones requires a diet that is abundant in calcium and vitamin D. Calcium is essential for strong bones, and vitamin D aids in its absorption by the body. Recent research highlights the significance of a well-rounded diet that incorporates magnesium, vitamin K, and proteins, in addition to the two mentioned nutrients, as they all play a role in promoting strong bones.

New research indicates that there are other nutrients and dietary patterns that play a role in maintaining strong bones. Take, for example, how certain diets and antioxidant-rich foods may help reduce the chances of developing osteoporosis. Furthermore, it is crucial to prioritize bone health by maintaining a healthy weight and limiting alcohol and caffeine intake.

HOW THIS COOKBOOK CAN HELP

This cookbook is created with the intention of being a helpful resource for individuals who have osteoporosis or those who want to take preventive measures against the condition. Every recipe is carefully created with a focus on the nutritional requirements necessary for promoting and enhancing bone health. The recipes are straightforward and cover a wide range of flavors and dietary needs, ensuring that even those new to cooking or with some experience can easily follow along.

In addition to providing mouthwatering, bone-strengthening recipes, this cookbook offers detailed information on osteoporosis. It incorporates up-to-date scientific research and insights from professionals in the field, making it a valuable resource for individuals seeking to gain a deeper understanding of the impact of diet on bone health. Whether you are a beginner in the kitchen or someone who wants to take charge of their bone health, this cookbook is designed to provide you with valuable information and delicious recipes that will nourish your body.

The "Osteoporosis Cookbook" goes beyond being a mere recipe collection. It is a complete guide that seamlessly blends delicious dishes with scientific insights, providing a well-rounded approach to managing osteoporosis through dietary choices.

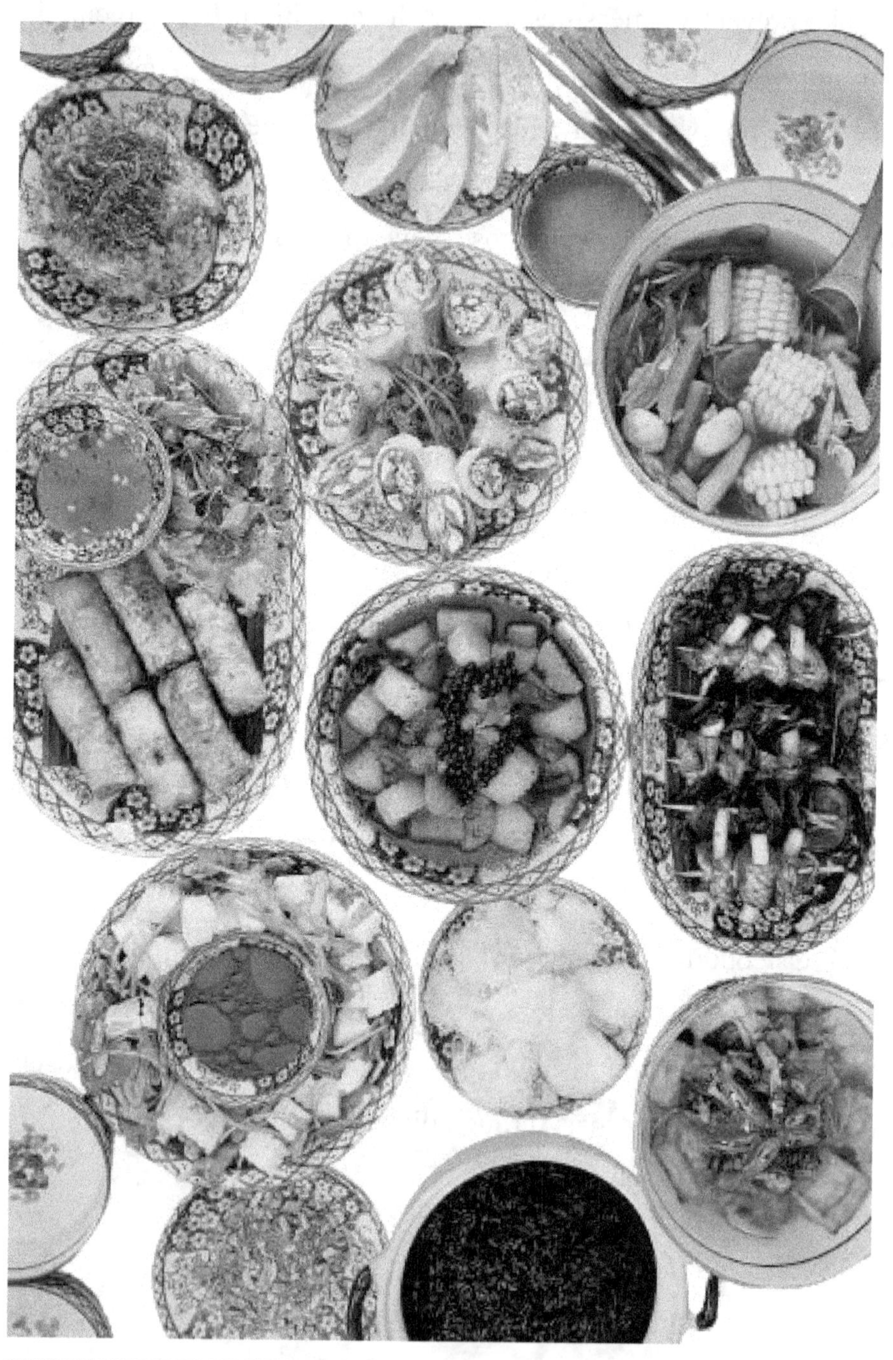

2. BUILDING STRONG BONES: A GUIDE TO PREVENTING OSTEOPOROSIS

ESSENTIAL NUTRIENTS FOR STRONGER BONES

Start your battle against osteoporosis with the power of nutrition. Several key nutrients are essential for maintaining strong and healthy bones:

1. Calcium: This is an incredibly important mineral when it comes to keeping your bones healthy. It plays a vital role in building and maintaining strong bones. For adults, the recommended dietary allowance (RDA) is 1,000 mg per day. However, women over 50 and men over 70 should aim for 1,200 mg per day. Calcium can be found in a variety of sources, including dairy products, leafy greens, almonds, and fortified foods.

2. Vitamin D: The main function of vitamin D is to assist the body in absorbing calcium. Insufficient vitamin D levels may result in weakened bones that are prone to breakage or deformity. For adults, the recommended daily allowance (RDA) is typically 600-

800 IU. However, some professionals recommend higher doses, particularly for individuals who may be at risk of deficiency. Getting enough vitamin D is essential for your health. You can find it in natural sources like sun exposure, as well as in fatty fish, fortified milk, and supplements.

<u>3. Magnesium and Potassium</u>: These minerals play a vital role in supporting bone health by aiding in bone formation and maintaining bone density. These foods are fantastic sources of nutrition.

<u>4. Protein</u>: This is crucial for maintaining strong and healthy bones. Research indicates that a diet lacking in sufficient protein can contribute to the weakening of bones, particularly among older individuals. Include sources such as lean meats, fish, dairy, beans, and nuts.

<u>5. Vitamins K and C</u>: These are important for maintaining healthy bones. Vitamin K helps with bone metabolism, while Vitamin C is necessary for producing collagen, which is a vital part of bone tissue. Leafy greens and citrus fruits are fantastic options.

Aside from the mentioned nutrients, there are certain dietary patterns that can be beneficial:

- *Mediterranean Diet:* Discover the wonders of the Mediterranean Diet, a nutritional approach that promotes strong bones and reduces the risk of fractures. This diet emphasizes the consumption of fruits, vegetables, nuts, olive oil, and fish.

- *Foods that Fight Inflammation:* Long-term inflammation can have a detrimental effect on the health of your bones. Certain foods, such as turmeric, ginger, fatty fish, and berries, have been found to have anti-inflammatory properties.

On the other hand, certain foods and substances can have a negative impact on bone health:

- *Excessive Salt:* Consuming too much salt can lead to increased calcium excretion through the kidneys.

- Caffeine and Alcohol: Excessive consumption of caffeine and alcohol can disrupt the absorption of calcium and negatively impact bone health.

BALANCING YOUR DIET FOR OPTIMAL BONE HEALTH

Incorporating Bone-Healthy Foods into Your Diet

Having a balanced diet is essential for maintaining strong bones, particularly for individuals who have osteoporosis or are prone to developing it. It goes beyond just eating the right nutrients; it's about incorporating them into your everyday meals in a manner that is both enjoyable and easy to sustain.

1. Mastering Portion Sizes: Grasping the right amount of each food group to consume is crucial. For example, a serving of dairy could be a cup of milk or yogurt, or an ounce of cheese. When it comes to vegetables and fruits, it's a good idea to aim for filling half your plate with these nutrient-rich options.

2. *Embrace Variety:* Incorporating a diverse selection of foods into your diet allows you to benefit from a wide array of essential nutrients. For instance, while dairy products are known for their calcium content, there are also other sources such as fortified plant milks, tofu, and leafy greens. Enhancing your overall nutrient intake can be achieved by diversifying your protein sources. This can include incorporating both animal and plant-based options such as beans and lentils.

3. *Cooking Methods Matter:* The manner in which you prepare your food can have an impact on its nutritional value. For example, when it comes to vegetables, steaming or roasting is a better option as it helps retain more nutrients compared to boiling. In comparison, opting for grilling fish or baking chicken is a healthier choice than frying.

CLEARING UP COMMON DIETARY MISCONCEPTIONS

Let's address some common myths and misconceptions about diet and bone health:

1. *Protein and Bone Health:* New research suggests that a higher protein diet, combined with sufficient calcium intake, can have positive effects on bone health, especially in older adults. It is no longer believed that excessive protein intake is harmful to bones.

2. ***There are alternative sources of calcium:*** Although dairy is commonly associated with calcium, it's important to note that many individuals are lactose intolerant or follow vegan diets. Include a variety of nutritious options like green leafy vegetables, almonds, sesame seeds, tofu, and fortified plant-based milks.

3. ***The role of acid and alkaline foods***: The notion that consuming alkaline foods, such as fruits and vegetables, instead of acidic foods like meat and dairy, can enhance bone health lacks substantial scientific support. It's crucial to prioritize a well-rounded diet rather than fixating solely on the pH of foods.

BEYOND DIET: LIFESTYLE CONSIDERATIONS FOR BONE HEALTH

While diet is important, there are other lifestyle factors that are also important for maintaining healthy bones:

1. ***Regular Exercise:*** Incorporating regular exercise into your routine is essential for building and maintaining bone density. It's

important to focus on weight-bearing and muscle-strengthening exercises.

2. ***Steer clear of smoking and keep alcohol intake in check:*** Smoking and drinking too much alcohol can have a negative impact on the health of your bones.

3. ***Stress Management:*** Long-term stress can cause hormonal imbalances that might affect bone density.

Simply put, the aim is to offer a comprehensive approach to bone health, blending cutting-edge scientific knowledge with practical tips for everyday life. This all-encompassing approach aims to empower individuals with osteoporosis to enhance their well-being and enhance their quality of life by making informed dietary and lifestyle choices.

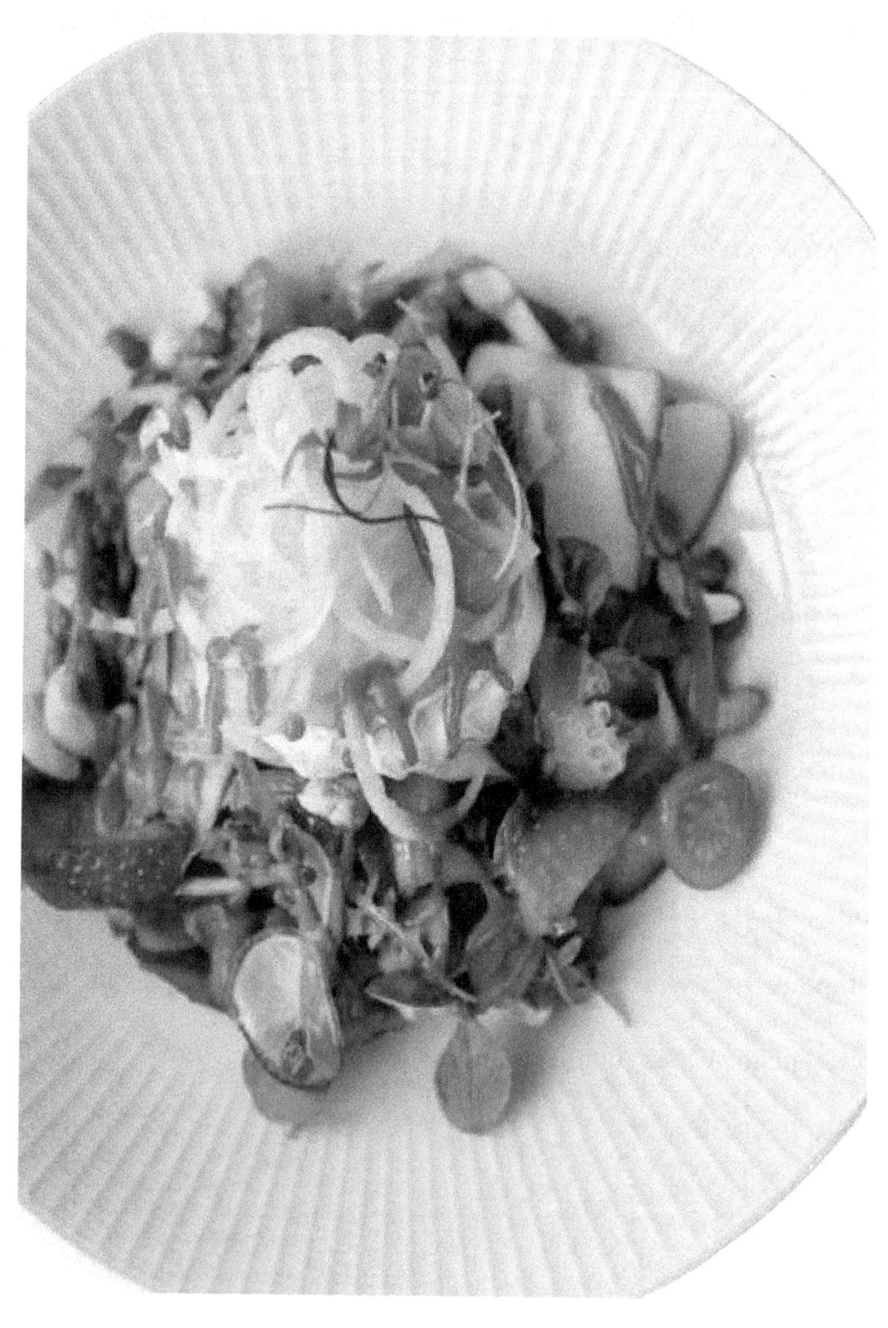

3. BREAKFAST RECIPES

1. Fortified Oatmeal Variations

Prep Time: 5 minutes || Cook Time: 10 minutes ||
Serving Size: 2 servings

Ingredients:

- 1 cup rolled oats

- 2 cups fortified almond milk (rich in calcium and vitamin D)

- 1 tbsp chia seeds (for omega-3s and fiber)

- 1 medium banana, sliced

- 2 tbsp almond slivers

- 1/4 tsp cinnamon

- 1 tbsp honey or maple syrup (optional)

Nutritional Content (per serving):

- Calories: 350 kcal

- Calcium: 30% of Daily Value (DV)

- Vitamin D: 25% DV

- Protein: 12g

- Fiber: 7g

Preparation Instructions:

1. Combine oats and fortified almond milk in a medium saucepan. Bring to a boil.
2. Reduce heat and simmer, stirring occasionally, for about 5-7 minutes.
3. Stir in chia seeds and cook for another 2-3 minutes until the mixture thickens.
4. Remove from heat. Add sliced banana, almond slivers, cinnamon, and honey/maple syrup if desired.
5. Serve warm.

Health Benefit:

This oatmeal is a great source of calcium and vitamin D, essential for bone health. The addition of chia seeds provides omega-3 fatty acids and fiber, supporting overall health and aiding in nutrient absorption, crucial for osteoporosis management.

Prep Time: 5 minutes || Cook Time: 0 minutes ||
Serving Size: 1 serving

Ingredients:

- 1 cup spinach (rich in calcium and vitamin K)

- 1/2 cup Greek yogurt (high in protein and calcium)

- 1/2 banana

- 1/4 cup mixed berries

- 1 tbsp ground flaxseed (for omega-3s)

- 1 cup fortified orange juice (for vitamin C and calcium)

Nutritional Content (per serving):

- Calories: 280 kcal

- Calcium: 35% DV

- Vitamin C: 100% DV

- Protein: 15g

- Fiber: 5g

Preparation Instructions:

1. Place spinach, Greek yogurt, banana, mixed berries, ground flaxseed, and fortified orange juice in a blender.

2. Blend on high speed until smooth.

3. Pour into a glass and enjoy immediately.

Health Benefit:

This smoothie is not only high in calcium and vitamin C but also rich in protein and fiber, providing a balanced, nutrient-dense start to the day. The inclusion of spinach and Greek yogurt boosts the calcium content, essential for strengthening bones.

3. Calcium-Rich Pancakes and Waffles

Prep Time: 10 minutes || Cook Time: 15 minutes || Serving Size: 4 servings

Ingredients:

- 1 1/2 cups whole wheat flour (for fiber)

- 1/2 cup almond flour (for calcium and protein)

- 2 tsp baking powder

- 1/4 tsp salt

- 2 eggs

- 1 1/4 cups fortified milk

- 2 tbsp melted unsalted butter

- 1 tsp vanilla extract

Nutritional Content (per serving):

- Calories: 330 kcal

- Calcium: 20% DV

- Protein: 12g

- Fiber: 4g

Preparation Instructions:

1. In a large bowl, mix together whole wheat flour, almond flour, baking powder, and salt.

2. In another bowl, whisk together eggs, fortified milk, melted butter, and vanilla extract.

3. Pour the wet ingredients into the dry ingredients and stir until just combined.

4. Heat a non-stick pan or waffle iron. Pour batter to form pancakes or waffles. Cook until golden brown.

5. Serve with fresh fruits and a drizzle of honey if desired.

Health Benefit:

These pancakes and waffles offer a great start to the day with a significant amount of calcium and protein, promoting bone strength and overall health. The use of whole wheat and almond flour adds fiber and additional nutrients beneficial for those managing osteoporosis.

Prep Time: 5 minutes || Cook Time: 5 minutes ||
Serving Size: 2 servings

Ingredients:

- 2 slices of whole grain bread (for fiber)

- 1 ripe avocado

- 2 eggs

- Pinch of salt and pepper

- 1 tbsp grated Parmesan cheese (for calcium)

Nutritional Content (per serving):

- Calories: 280 kcal

- Calcium: 15% DV

- Protein: 12g

- Fiber: 6g

Preparation Instructions:

1. Toast the whole grain bread slices.

2. Mash the avocado and spread it on the toast.

3. Fry or poach the eggs and place them on top of the avocado.

4. Season with salt and pepper, and sprinkle with Parmesan cheese.

5. Serve immediately.

Health Benefit:

This recipe offers a balance of healthy fats, protein, and fiber. The avocado provides beneficial fats, while the Parmesan adds a good calcium boost, which is crucial for bone health in osteoporosis management.

5. Spinach and Feta Omelette

Prep Time: 5 minutes || Cook Time: 10 minutes ||
Serving Size: 1 serving

Ingredients:

- 2 eggs

- 1 cup fresh spinach (for vitamin K and calcium)

- 1/4 cup crumbled feta cheese (for calcium)

- 1 tbsp olive oil

- Salt and pepper to taste

Nutritional Content (per serving):

- Calories: 320 kcal

- Calcium: 25% DV

- Protein: 18g

- Fiber: 2g

Preparation Instructions:

1. Beat the eggs in a bowl. Season with salt and pepper.

2. Heat olive oil in a pan. Sauté spinach until wilted.

3. Pour the beaten eggs over the spinach. Sprinkle feta cheese on top.

4. Cook until the eggs are set, then fold the omelette in half.

5. Serve hot.

Health Benefit:

This omelette is rich in calcium from the feta cheese and spinach, which is vital for bone health. The high protein content from the eggs aids in muscle maintenance, important for overall health in osteoporosis patients.

6. Quinoa Breakfast Bowl

Prep Time: 5 minutes (if using pre-cooked quinoa) || Cook Time: 15 minutes || Serving Size: 2 servings

Ingredients:

- 1 cup cooked quinoa (for protein and magnesium)

- 1/2 cup blueberries

- 1/4 cup chopped nuts (almonds, walnuts)

- 1 tbsp chia seeds

- 1 cup almond milk, fortified

- 1 tbsp honey or maple syrup

Nutritional Content (per serving):

- Calories: 360 kcal

- Calcium: 20% DV

- Protein: 10g

- Fiber: 7g

Preparation Instructions:

1. In a bowl, combine cooked quinoa with almond milk.

2. Top with blueberries, chopped nuts, and chia seeds.

3. Drizzle with honey or maple syrup.

4. Serve either hot or cold.

Health Benefit:

Quinoa is a complete protein and rich in magnesium, important for bone health. The addition of chia seeds and nuts provides omega-3 fatty acids and additional calcium, enhancing the osteoporosis-fighting capabilities of this meal.

Prep Time: 5 minutes || Serving Size: 1 serving

Ingredients:

- 1 cup Greek yogurt (rich in calcium and protein)

- 1/2 cup mixed berries (strawberries, blueberries, raspberries)

- 1 tbsp honey or maple syrup

- 2 tbsp granola (for added fiber and crunch)

Nutritional Content (per serving):

- Calories: 250 kcal

- Calcium: 30% DV

- Protein: 20g

- Fiber: 3g

Preparation Instructions:

1. Pour Greek yogurt into a bowl.

2. Top with mixed berries.

3. Drizzle with honey or maple syrup.

4. Sprinkle granola on top.

5. Serve and enjoy.

Health Benefit:

Greek yogurt is an excellent source of calcium and protein, which are essential for bone health. Berries add antioxidants and additional vitamins, making this an ideal breakfast for those managing osteoporosis.

8. Almond Butter and Banana Smoothie

Prep Time: 5 minutes || Serving Size: 1 serving

Ingredients:

- 1 banana

- 2 tbsp almond butter (for healthy fats and calcium)

- 1 cup fortified soy milk (for calcium and vitamin D)

- 1/2 tsp vanilla extract

- Ice cubes (optional)

Nutritional Content (per serving):

- Calories: 320 kcal

- Calcium: 25% DV

- Protein: 10g

- Fiber: 4g

Preparation Instructions:

1. Place banana, almond butter, fortified soy milk, and vanilla extract in a blender.

2. Add ice cubes if a colder smoothie is desired.

3. Blend until smooth.

4. Serve immediately.

Health Benefit:

Almond butter is a good source of calcium and healthy fats, which are beneficial for bone health. The soy milk adds extra calcium and vitamin D, making this smoothie a nutritious choice for osteoporosis management.

9. Kale and Mushroom Breakfast Saute

Prep Time: 10 minutes || Cook Time: 10 minutes ||
Serving Size: 2 servings

Ingredients:

- 2 cups chopped kale (rich in calcium and vitamin K)

- 1 cup sliced mushrooms

- 2 cloves garlic, minced

- 2 tbsp olive oil

- Salt and pepper to taste

- 2 tbsp grated Parmesan cheese

Nutritional Content (per serving):

- Calories: 180 kcal

- Calcium: 20% DV

- Protein: 6g

- Fiber: 3g

Preparation Instructions:

1. Heat olive oil in a pan over medium heat.
2. Add garlic and mushrooms; sauté until mushrooms are golden.
3. Add kale and cook until wilted.
4. Season with salt and pepper.
5. Sprinkle with Parmesan cheese before serving.

Health Benefit:

Kale is one of the best plant-based sources of calcium, and mushrooms provide additional nutrients. This sauté is a great way to start the day with a high-calcium, bone-healthy meal.

Prep Time: 5 minutes || Serving Size: 1 serving

Ingredients:

- 1 cup cottage cheese (high in calcium and protein)

- 1/2 cup chopped pineapple (for vitamin C)

- 1 tbsp sliced almonds

- 1 tsp honey (optional)

Nutritional Content (per serving):

- Calories: 220 kcal

- Calcium: 20% DV

- Protein: 25g

- Fiber: 2g

Preparation Instructions:

1. Place cottage cheese in a bowl.

2. Top with chopped pineapple and sliced almonds.

3. Drizzle with honey if desired.

4. Serve and enjoy.

Health Benefit:

Cottage cheese is an excellent source of calcium and protein, which are vital for bone health. Pineapple adds a burst of vitamin C, enhancing the overall nutritional profile of this osteoporosis-friendly breakfast.

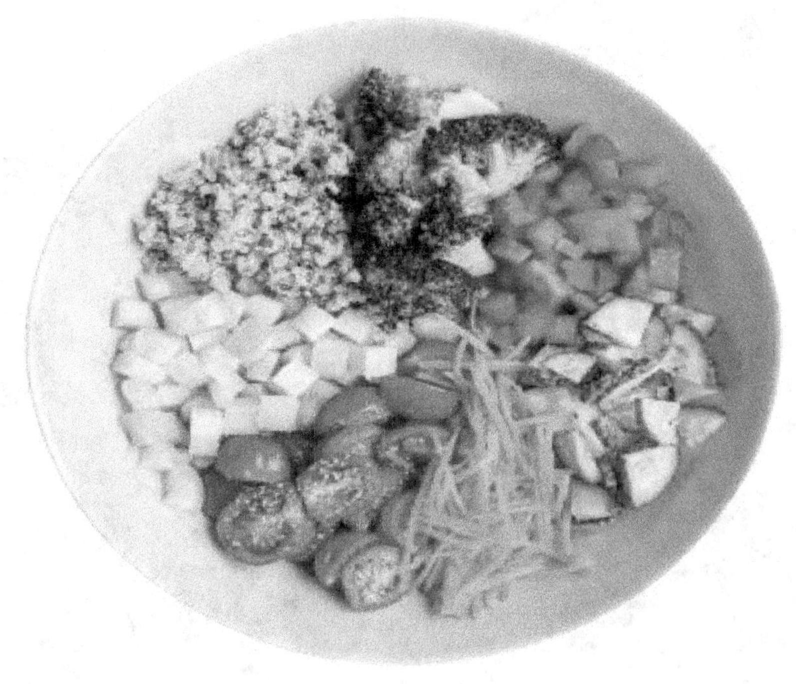

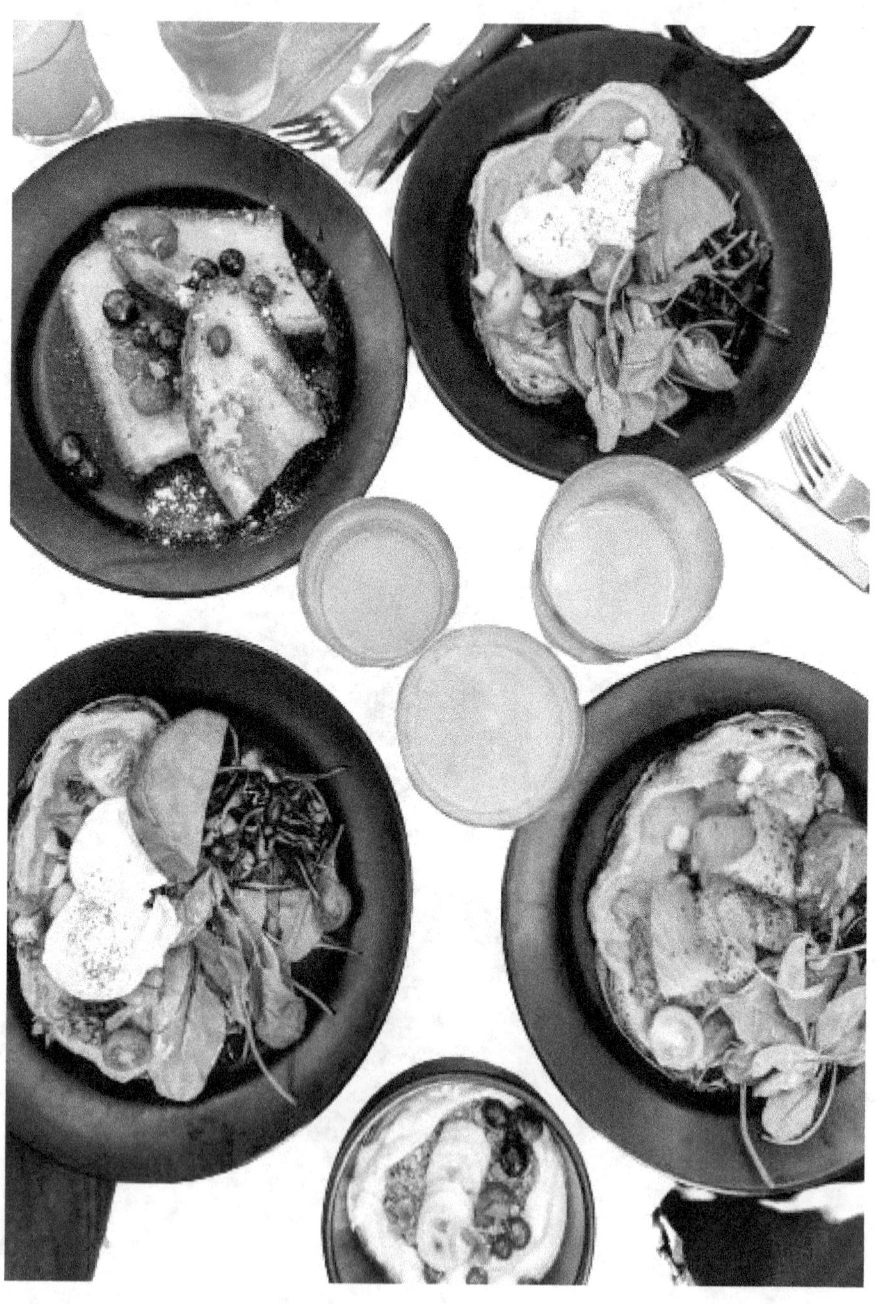

4. LUNCH RECIPES

11. Hearty Salmon Salad

***Prep Time: 10 minutes || Cook Time: 15 minutes ||
Serving Size: 2 servings***

Ingredients:

- 2 salmon fillets (rich in omega-3 fatty acids)
- 4 cups mixed greens (spinach, arugula, and kale for calcium and vitamin K)
- 1/2 avocado, sliced
- 1/4 cup cherry tomatoes, halved
- 1/4 cup cucumber, sliced
- 2 tbsp olive oil
- 1 tbsp lemon juice
- Salt and pepper to taste

Nutritional Content (per serving):

- Calories: 380 kcal
- Calcium: 15% DV
- Omega-3 fatty acids: High
- Protein: 24g
- Fiber: 4g

1. Season salmon fillets with salt and pepper. Grill or pan-sear until cooked.
2. Mix mixed greens, avocado, cherry tomatoes, and cucumber in a bowl.
3. Whisk together olive oil and lemon juice, drizzle over the salad.
4. Top salad with cooked salmon.
5. Serve immediately.

Health Benefit:

Rich in omega-3 fatty acids, this salmon salad is excellent for bone health. The leafy greens add a significant amount of calcium and vitamin K, which are crucial for strengthening bones and managing osteoporosis.

12. Quinoa and Black Bean Bowl

Prep Time: 10 minutes || Cook Time: 20 minutes ||
Serving Size: 2 servings

Ingredients:

- 1 cup cooked quinoa (for protein and magnesium)
- 1/2 cup black beans (for protein and fiber)

- 1/2 cup corn kernels

- 1/2 red bell pepper, diced

- 1/4 cup fresh cilantro, chopped

- 2 tbsp lime juice

- 1 tbsp olive oil

- Salt and pepper to taste

Nutritional Content (per serving):

- Calories: 350 kcal

- Calcium: 10% DV

- Protein: 12g

- Fiber: 7g

Preparation Instructions:

1. Combine cooked quinoa, black beans, corn, and red bell pepper in a bowl.
2. In a small bowl, whisk together lime juice, olive oil, salt, and pepper.
3. Pour the dressing over the quinoa mixture and toss well.
4. Garnish with fresh cilantro.
5. Serve either warm or cold.

<u>***Health Benefit:***</u>

Quinoa is a complete protein and rich in magnesium, important for bone health. Black beans add additional protein and fiber, enhancing the overall nutritional value of this meal for osteoporosis management.

13. Tofu and Vegetable Stir-Fry

Prep Time: 10 minutes || Cook Time: 10 minutes || Serving Size: 2 servings

Ingredients:

- 1 block firm tofu, cubed (rich in calcium and protein)
- 2 cups mixed vegetables (broccoli, carrots, bell peppers)
- 2 tbsp soy sauce (low sodium)
- 1 tbsp sesame oil
- 1 tsp ginger, grated
- 1 garlic clove, minced
- Sesame seeds for garnish

Nutritional Content (per serving):

- Calories: 320 kcal
- Calcium: 20% DV
- Protein: 18g
- Fiber: 4g

Preparation Instructions:

1. Press tofu to remove excess water and cut into cubes.

2. Heat sesame oil in a pan, add ginger and garlic, and sauté for a minute.

3. Add mixed vegetables and stir-fry until crisp-tender.

4. Add tofu and soy sauce, cook for another 5 minutes.

5. Garnish with sesame seeds before serving.

Health Benefit:

Tofu is a great source of calcium, making it an excellent choice for bone health. The mixed vegetables contribute additional nutrients and fiber, essential for a balanced diet in osteoporosis management.

14. Chicken Caesar Salad Wrap

Prep Time: 15 minutes || Cook Time: 10 minutes ||
Serving Size: 2 servings

Ingredients:

- 2 whole grain wraps

- 1 grilled chicken breast, sliced (for protein)

- 2 cups romaine lettuce, chopped

- 1/4 cup Caesar dressing, low-fat

- 2 tbsp Parmesan cheese, grated

- 1/4 cup croutons, whole grain

<u>**Nutritional Content (per serving):**</u>

- Calories: 400 kcal

- Calcium: 15% DV

- Protein: 25g

- Fiber: 5g

<u>**Preparation Instructions:**</u>

1. Lay out the whole grain wraps.

2. Distribute romaine lettuce and grilled chicken slices evenly on each wrap.

3. Drizzle with Caesar dressing and sprinkle with Parmesan cheese.

4. Add croutons for crunch.

5. Roll up the wraps tightly and cut in half.

6. Serve immediately.

<u>**Health Benefit:**</u>

This wrap provides a good balance of protein from chicken and calcium from the Parmesan cheese, both important for bone health. The whole grain wrap adds fiber, aiding in overall digestive health.

Prep Time: 10 minutes || Serving Size: 2 servings

Ingredients:

- 1 can chickpeas, drained and rinsed (for protein and fiber)

- 1/2 cucumber, diced

- 1/2 red onion, finely chopped

- 1/4 cup Kalamata olives, sliced

- 1/4 cup feta cheese, crumbled (for calcium)

- 2 tbsp olive oil

- 1 tbsp lemon juice

- Salt and pepper to taste

Nutritional Content (per serving):

- Calories: 360 kcal

- Calcium: 15% DV

- Protein: 12g

- Fiber: 6g

1. In a bowl, combine chickpeas, cucumber, red onion, olives, and feta cheese.
2. In a small bowl, whisk together olive oil, lemon juice, salt, and pepper.
3. Pour the dressing over the salad and toss well.
4. Serve chilled or at room temperature.

<u>**Health Benefit:**</u>

Chickpeas are a great source of protein and fiber, and feta cheese adds a healthy dose of calcium. This salad is not only nutritious but also aligns with a Mediterranean diet, which is beneficial for bone health.

16. Broccoli and Cheese Stuffed Baked Potato

Prep Time: 5 minutes || Cook Time: 45 minutes (for baking potato) || Serving Size: 2 servings

<u>**Ingredients:**</u>

- 2 large baking potatoes
- 1 cup broccoli florets, steamed (rich in calcium and vitamin K)
- 1/2 cup cheddar cheese, shredded (for calcium)
- 2 tbsp Greek yogurt (for added protein and creaminess)
- Salt and pepper to taste

<u>**Nutritional Content (per serving):**</u>

- Calories: 350 kcal

- Calcium: 25% DV

- Protein: 15g

- Fiber: 6g

<u>**Preparation Instructions:**</u>

1. Preheat the oven to 400°F (200°C). Pierce potatoes with a fork and bake until tender, about 45 minutes.
2. Cut a slit in each potato and scoop out some of the flesh to make a small "bowl."
3. Mix the scooped potato flesh with steamed broccoli, cheddar cheese, Greek yogurt, salt, and pepper.
4. Stuff this mixture back into the potato skins.
5. Bake for an additional 10 minutes until the cheese is melted.
6. Serve hot.

<u>**Health Benefit:**</u>

This dish is a comforting, calcium-rich meal. Broccoli and cheddar cheese provide a good dose of calcium, while the potato adds fiber and other essential nutrients, making it an excellent choice for bone health.

Prep Time: 10 minutes || Cook Time: 30 minutes ||
Serving Size: 3 servings

Ingredients:

- 1 cup lentils (for protein and fiber)

- 1 onion, chopped

- 2 carrots, diced

- 2 cups spinach (for calcium and vitamin K)

- 4 cups vegetable broth

- 2 tbsp olive oil

- 1 tsp cumin

- Salt and pepper to taste

Nutritional Content (per serving):

- Calories: 250 kcal

- Calcium: 15% DV

- Protein: 15g

- Fiber: 8g

Preparation Instructions:

1. Heat olive oil in a pot. Add onion and carrots, sauté until soft.

2. Add lentils, cumin, salt, pepper, and vegetable broth.

3. Bring to a boil, then simmer for 20 minutes until lentils are tender.

4. Stir in spinach and cook until wilted.

5. Serve hot.

Health Benefit:

Lentils are an excellent protein and fiber source, aiding in bone and overall health. The addition of spinach boosts the calcium and vitamin K content, making this soup a hearty and nutritious option for those managing osteoporosis.

18. Turkey and Avocado Wrap

Prep Time: 5 minutes || Serving Size: 2 servings

Ingredients:

- 2 whole grain wraps

- 4 slices of turkey breast (for lean protein)

- 1 ripe avocado, sliced

- 1 cup baby spinach (for calcium and vitamin K)

- 1/4 cup shredded carrot

- 2 tbsp hummus

- Salt and pepper to taste

<u>**Nutritional Content (per serving):**</u>

- Calories: 380 kcal

- Calcium: 10% DV

- Protein: 20g

- Fiber: 6g

<u>**Preparation Instructions:**</u>

1. Spread hummus evenly on the whole grain wraps.
2. Lay turkey slices over the hummus.
3. Add sliced avocado, baby spinach, and shredded carrot on top of the turkey.
4. Season with salt and pepper.
5. Roll up the wraps tightly and cut in half.
6. Serve immediately.

<u>**Health Benefit:**</u>

This wrap is a great source of lean protein from the turkey and healthy fats from the avocado. The spinach adds calcium and vitamin K, making it an excellent lunch choice for managing osteoporosis.

Prep Time: 10 minutes || Cook Time: 30 minutes ||
Serving Size: 4 servings

Ingredients:

- 2 medium sweet potatoes, peeled and diced

- 1 can black beans, drained and rinsed (for protein and fiber)

- 1 onion, chopped

- 2 garlic cloves, minced

- 1 can diced tomatoes

- 2 cups vegetable broth

- 1 tbsp chili powder

- 1 tsp cumin

- 2 tbsp olive oil

- Salt and pepper to taste

Nutritional Content (per serving):

- Calories: 300 kcal

- Calcium: 10% DV

- Protein: 8g

- Fiber: 9g

<u>**Preparation Instructions:**</u>

1. Heat olive oil in a large pot. Add onion and garlic, sauté until soft.
2. Add sweet potatoes, black beans, diced tomatoes, vegetable broth, chili powder, and cumin.
3. Bring to a boil, then reduce heat and simmer for 25-30 minutes until sweet potatoes are tender.
4. Season with salt and pepper.
5. Serve hot.

<u>**Health Benefit:**</u>

Sweet potatoes are high in vitamin C and beneficial for bone health. Combined with protein-rich black beans, this chili is not only hearty and filling but also beneficial for maintaining bone strength.

20. Greek-Style Stuffed Bell Peppers

Prep Time: 15 minutes || Cook Time: 30 minutes ||
Serving Size: 4 servings

<u>**Ingredients:**</u>

- 4 bell peppers, tops cut off and seeded
- 1 cup cooked quinoa

- 1/2 cup feta cheese, crumbled (for calcium)

- 1 cup spinach, chopped (for calcium and vitamin K)

- 1/4 cup Kalamata olives, chopped

- 2 tbsp olive oil

- 1 tsp dried oregano

- Salt and pepper to taste

Nutritional Content (per serving):

- Calories: 280 kcal

- Calcium: 15% DV

- Protein: 8g

- Fiber: 5g

Preparation Instructions:

1. Preheat oven to 375°F (190°C).
2. In a bowl, mix quinoa, feta cheese, spinach, Kalamata olives, olive oil, oregano, salt, and pepper.
3. Stuff this mixture into the bell peppers.
4. Place stuffed peppers in a baking dish and bake for 30 minutes until peppers are tender.
5. Serve hot.

<u>Health Benefit:</u>

Bell peppers are high in vitamin C, which is important for collagen formation in bones. The addition of quinoa and feta cheese provides protein and calcium, enhancing the dish's benefits for bone health.

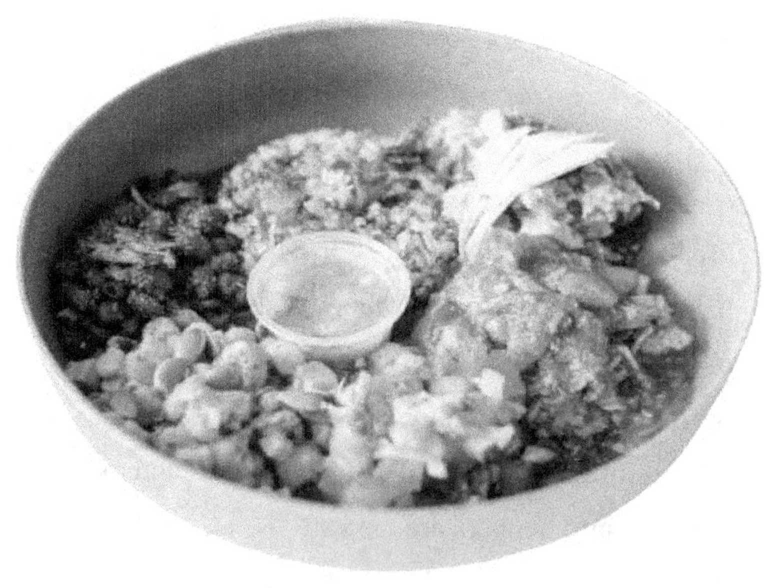

5. DINNER RECIPES

21. Baked Lemon-Garlic Salmon

Prep Time: 5 minutes || Cook Time: 20 minutes ||
Serving Size: 2 servings

Ingredients:

- 2 salmon fillets (rich in omega-3 fatty acids)

- 2 garlic cloves, minced

- 1 lemon, juiced and zested

- 2 tbsp olive oil

- Salt and pepper to taste

- Fresh dill for garnish

Nutritional Content (per serving):

- Calories: 370 kcal

- Omega-3 fatty acids: High

- Protein: 34g

- Calcium: 5% DV

<u>***Preparation Instructions:***</u>

1. Preheat oven to 375°F (190°C).
2. Place salmon fillets in a baking dish.
3. Mix lemon juice, zest, garlic, olive oil, salt, and pepper. Pour over salmon.
4. Bake for 15-20 minutes, until salmon flakes easily.
5. Garnish with fresh dill and serve.

<u>***Health Benefit:***</u>

Salmon is an excellent source of omega-3 fatty acids, which are known to enhance bone health. The lemon adds a dose of vitamin C, aiding in collagen formation for strong bones.

22. Grilled Chicken and Vegetable Kabobs

Prep Time: 15 minutes (plus marinating time) || Cook Time: 10 minutes || Serving Size: 4 servings

<u>***Ingredients:***</u>

- 2 boneless chicken breasts, cut into cubes

- 1 zucchini, sliced

- 1 red bell pepper, cut into pieces

- 1 yellow bell pepper, cut into pieces

- 1 onion, cut into wedges

- 2 tbsp olive oil

- 1 tbsp balsamic vinegar

- 1 garlic clove, minced

- 1 tsp dried Italian herbs

- Salt and pepper to taste

Nutritional Content (per serving):

- Calories: 220 kcal

- Protein: 26g

- Calcium: 3% DV

- Fiber: 2g

Preparation Instructions:

1. Whisk together olive oil, balsamic vinegar, garlic, Italian herbs, salt, and pepper. Marinate chicken pieces in this mixture for at least 30 minutes.

2. Thread chicken, zucchini, bell peppers, and onion onto skewers.

3. Grill over medium heat for 10 minutes, turning occasionally, until chicken is cooked through.

4. Serve hot.

Health Benefit:

This dish is high in protein from chicken and rich in vitamins from the colorful vegetables. Protein is essential for bone repair and maintenance, making this a great choice for osteoporosis management.

Prep Time: 10 minutes || Cook Time: 40 minutes ||
Serving Size: 2 servings

Ingredients:

- 1 acorn squash, halved and seeded
- 1 cup quinoa, cooked
- 1/4 cup cranberries
- 1/4 cup chopped walnuts
- 1/4 cup feta cheese, crumbled
- 2 tbsp maple syrup
- 1 tsp cinnamon
- Salt and pepper to taste
- Olive oil

Nutritional Content (per serving):

- Calories: 450 kcal
- Calcium: 10% DV
- Protein: 10g
- Fiber: 6g

<u>**Preparation Instructions:**</u>

1. Preheat oven to 375°F (190°C).

2. Brush acorn squash halves with olive oil, season with salt and pepper. Place cut-side down on a baking sheet and roast for 25 minutes.

3. Mix cooked quinoa, cranberries, walnuts, feta cheese, maple syrup, and cinnamon.

4. Turn squash halves cut-side up and fill with quinoa mixture.

5. Roast for an additional 15 minutes.

6. Serve warm.

<u>**Health Benefit:**</u>

Acorn squash is high in fiber and antioxidants. Quinoa adds protein, and walnuts provide healthy fats, making this a well-rounded, nutritious meal for bone health.

Prep Time: 10 minutes || Cook Time: 10 minutes ||
Serving Size: 2 servings

Ingredients:

- 1 block firm tofu, cubed

- 2 cups broccoli florets

- 1 red bell pepper, sliced

- 2 tbsp soy sauce (low sodium)

- 1 tbsp sesame oil

- 1 garlic clove, minced

- 1 tsp ginger, grated

- Sesame seeds for garnish

Nutritional Content (per serving):

- Calories: 320 kcal

- Calcium: 25% DV

- Protein: 18g

- Fiber: 4g

<u>**Preparation Instructions:**</u>

1. Press tofu to remove excess water, then cut into cubes.

2. Heat sesame oil in a pan, add garlic and ginger, sauté for a minute.

3. Add tofu, broccoli, and red bell pepper. Stir-fry for 5 minutes.

4. Add soy sauce, stir well, and cook for another 5 minutes.

5. Garnish with sesame seeds and serve.

<u>**Health Benefit:**</u>

Tofu is a fantastic source of calcium and protein, essential for bone health. Broccoli adds additional vitamins and minerals, enhancing the dish's overall nutritional value for osteoporosis management.

25. Lentil and Vegetable Stew

Prep Time: 10 minutes || Cook Time: 30 minutes ||
Serving Size: 4 servings

Ingredients:

- 1 cup lentils

- 1 onion, chopped

- 2 carrots, diced

- 2 potatoes, diced

- 4 cups vegetable broth

- 1 can diced tomatoes

- 2 tsp dried thyme

- Salt and pepper to taste

- 2 tbsp olive oil

Nutritional Content (per serving):

- Calories: 300 kcal

- Calcium: 5% DV

- Protein: 14g

- Fiber: 9g

<u>Preparation Instructions:</u>

1. Heat olive oil in a pot, add onion and carrots, cook until soft.
2. Add potatoes, lentils, diced tomatoes, vegetable broth, thyme, salt, and pepper.
3. Bring to a boil, reduce heat and simmer for 30 minutes until lentils and vegetables are tender.
4. Serve hot.

<u>Health Benefit:</u>

Lentils are rich in protein and fiber, contributing to bone and overall health. The vegetables add essential nutrients and antioxidants, making this stew a hearty and beneficial meal for osteoporosis management.

Prep Time: 15 minutes || Cook Time: 15 minutes ||
Serving Size: 2 servings

Ingredients:

- 1 block firm tofu, sliced

- 1 cup quinoa, cooked

- 2 tbsp lemon juice

- 1 tbsp olive oil

- 1 garlic clove, minced

- 1 tsp dried herbs (thyme, oregano)

- Salt and pepper to taste

- Fresh parsley for garnish

<u>**Nutritional Content (per serving):**</u>

- Calories: 350 kcal

- Calcium: 20% DV

- Protein: 20g

- Fiber: 5g

<u>*Preparation Instructions:*</u>

1. Marinate tofu slices in a mixture of lemon juice, olive oil, garlic, herbs, salt, and pepper for 30 minutes.
2. Grill tofu on medium heat until golden brown, about 5 minutes per side.
3. Serve grilled tofu over lemon herb quinoa.
4. Garnish with fresh parsley.

<u>*Health Benefit:*</u>

Tofu is an excellent source of calcium, essential for bone health. Quinoa adds protein and fiber, making this a balanced and nutritious meal for osteoporosis management.

27. Baked Cod with Tomato and Olive Tapenade

Prep Time: 10 minutes || Cook Time: 20 minutes || Serving Size: 2 servings

<u>*Ingredients:*</u>

- 2 cod fillets

- 1 cup cherry tomatoes, halved

- 1/4 cup Kalamata olives, chopped

- 1 tbsp olive oil

- 1 tsp lemon zest

- Salt and pepper to taste

- Fresh basil for garnish

Nutritional Content (per serving):

- Calories: 250 kcal

- Omega-3 fatty acids: High

- Protein: 22g

- Calcium: 3% DV

Preparation Instructions:

1. Preheat oven to 375°F (190°C).
2. Place cod fillets in a baking dish.
3. Mix tomatoes, olives, olive oil, lemon zest, salt, and pepper. Spoon over cod.
4. Bake for 20 minutes, until cod is flaky.
5. Garnish with fresh basil and serve.

Health Benefit:

Cod is a low-fat protein source, beneficial for maintaining a healthy weight. The omega-3 fatty acids in cod are important for bone health, and the tomatoes add a good dose of antioxidants.

Prep Time: 15 minutes || Cook Time: 30 minutes || Serving Size: 2 servings

Ingredients:

- 2 chicken breasts

- 1 cup ricotta cheese (for calcium)

- 1 cup spinach, chopped (for calcium and vitamin K)

- 1 garlic clove, minced

- Salt and pepper to taste

- 1 tbsp olive oil

Nutritional Content (per serving):

- Calories: 360 kcal

- Calcium: 20% DV

- Protein: 35g

- Fiber: 2g

Preparation Instructions:

1. Preheat oven to 375°F (190°C).

2. Make a horizontal cut in each chicken breast to create a pocket.

3. In a bowl, mix ricotta, spinach, garlic, salt, and pepper.

4. Stuff each chicken breast with the ricotta mixture.

5. Heat olive oil in a pan over medium heat, sear the chicken on both sides until golden.

6. Transfer to the oven and bake for 20 minutes, or until cooked through.

7. Serve hot.

Health Benefit:

This recipe combines high-quality protein from chicken with calcium from ricotta and spinach, making it an excellent dish for maintaining bone strength in osteoporosis management.

29. Butternut Squash Risotto

Prep Time: 10 minutes || Cook Time: 30 minutes ||
Serving Size: 4 servings

Ingredients:

- 1 butternut squash, peeled and cubed

- 1 cup Arborio rice

- 4 cups vegetable broth

- 1 onion, chopped

- 2 cloves garlic, minced

- 1/2 cup Parmesan cheese, grated (for calcium)

- 2 tbsp olive oil

- Salt and pepper to taste

Nutritional Content (per serving):

- Calories: 400 kcal

- Calcium: 10% DV

- Protein: 8g

- Fiber: 4g

Preparation Instructions:

1. Heat olive oil in a large pan, sauté onion and garlic until soft.
2. Add Arborio rice, stir for 2 minutes.
3. Gradually add vegetable broth, stirring constantly until absorbed, about 20 minutes.
4. In a separate pan, cook butternut squash until tender.
5. Mix cooked squash into the risotto.
6. Stir in Parmesan cheese, season with salt and pepper.
7. Serve warm.

<u>**Health Benefit:**</u>

Butternut squash is rich in vitamins A and C, beneficial for bone health. The addition of Parmesan cheese provides calcium, making this dish a healthy choice for individuals managing osteoporosis.

30. Grilled Vegetable and Halloumi Skewers

Prep Time: 15 minutes || Cook Time: 10 minutes ||
Serving Size: 4 servings

<u>**Ingredients:**</u>
- 1 block halloumi cheese, cubed (rich in calcium)
- 1 zucchini, sliced
- 1 red bell pepper, cut into pieces
- 1 yellow bell pepper, cut into pieces
- 1 red onion, cut into wedges
- 2 tbsp olive oil
- 1 tbsp lemon juice
- 1 tsp dried oregano
- Salt and pepper to taste

<u>**Nutritional Content (per serving):**</u>
- Calories: 300 kcal
- Calcium: 20% DV

- Protein: 12g

- Fiber: 3g

Preparation Instructions:

1. Preheat grill to medium heat.

2. Thread halloumi, zucchini, bell peppers, and onion onto skewers.

3. Whisk together olive oil, lemon juice, oregano, salt, and pepper.

4. Brush this mixture over the skewers.

5. Grill for 10 minutes, turning occasionally, until vegetables are tender and halloumi is golden brown.

6. Serve hot.

Health Benefit:

Halloumi is a high-calcium cheese, and when combined with vitamin-rich vegetables, these skewers make a delicious and bone-health-friendly meal, perfect for osteoporosis management.

6. SNACKS AND SMALL BITES

31. Greek Yogurt and Mixed Berry Parfait

Prep Time: 5 minutes || Serving Size: 1 serving

Ingredients:

- 1 cup Greek yogurt (rich in calcium and protein)

- 1/2 cup mixed berries (for antioxidants)

- 2 tbsp granola (for crunch and fiber)

- 1 tsp honey (optional)

Nutritional Content (per serving):

- Calories: 250 kcal

- Calcium: 25% DV

- Protein: 20g

- Fiber: 3g

Preparation Instructions:

1. Layer Greek yogurt, mixed berries, and granola in a glass or bowl.

2. Drizzle with honey if desired.

3. Serve immediately or refrigerate for a chilled snack.

Health Benefit:

Greek yogurt provides a high amount of calcium and protein, vital for bone health. The berries add antioxidants, while the granola offers fiber, making this a nutritious snack for osteoporosis management.

32. Almond and Date Energy Balls

Prep Time: 15 minutes || Serving Size: 10 balls

Ingredients:

- 1 cup dates, pitted
- 1/2 cup almonds (rich in calcium and healthy fats)
- 1/4 cup unsweetened shredded coconut
- 1 tbsp chia seeds (for omega-3s)
- 1 tsp vanilla extract

Nutritional Content (per ball):
- Calories: 100 kcal
- Calcium: 3% DV
- Protein: 2g
- Fiber: 2g

Preparation Instructions:

1. In a food processor, blend dates and almonds until a sticky dough forms.
2. Add shredded coconut, chia seeds, and vanilla extract, blend until mixed.
3. Roll the mixture into small balls.
4. Refrigerate for an hour before serving.

Health Benefit:

Almonds are a great source of calcium and healthy fats. Dates provide natural sweetness and energy, while chia seeds add omega-3 fatty acids, beneficial for bone health.

33. Baked Kale Chips

Prep Time: 10 minutes || Cook Time: 15 minutes ||
Serving Size: 2 servings

Ingredients:

- 1 bunch kale, stems removed and leaves torn

- 1 tbsp olive oil

- Salt to taste

Nutritional Content (per serving):

- Calories: 80 kcal

- Calcium: 10% DV

- Fiber: 2g

- Protein: 3g

Preparation Instructions:

1. Preheat oven to 300°F (150°C).

2. Toss kale leaves with olive oil and salt.

3. Spread on a baking sheet and bake for 15 minutes, until crisp.

4. Serve immediately.

Health Benefit:

Kale is a superfood, high in calcium and vitamins essential for bone health. Baked kale chips are a healthy, low-calorie alternative to traditional snacks.

34. Hummus and Veggie Sticks

Prep Time: 10 minutes || Serving Size: 2 servings

Ingredients:

- 1 cup hummus (rich in protein and fiber)

- 1 carrot, cut into sticks

- 1 cucumber, cut into sticks

- 1 red bell pepper, cut into sticks

Nutritional Content (per serving):

- Calories: 180 kcal

- Calcium: 5% DV

- Protein: 6g

- Fiber: 4g

Preparation Instructions:

1. Arrange hummus in a serving bowl.

2. Serve with carrot, cucumber, and bell pepper sticks.

3. Dip and enjoy.

Health Benefit:

Hummus, made from chickpeas, provides protein and fiber. The fresh vegetables offer vitamins and minerals, making this a healthy, bone-friendly snack option.

35. Cottage Cheese with Pineapple

Prep Time: 5 minutes || Serving Size: 1 serving

Ingredients:

- 1 cup cottage cheese (high in protein and calcium)

- 1/2 cup chopped pineapple (for vitamin C)

Nutritional Content (per serving):

- Calories: 220 kcal

- Calcium: 15% DV

- Protein: 25g

- Fiber: 1g

Preparation Instructions:

1. Place cottage cheese in a bowl.

2. Top with chopped pineapple.

3. Serve immediately.

Health Benefit:

Cottage cheese is an excellent source of calcium and protein. Pineapple adds vitamin C, enhancing the overall nutritional value of this snack for osteoporosis management.

36. Avocado Toast with Sesame Seeds

Prep Time: 5 minutes || Cook Time: 2 minutes (toasting bread)
Serving Size: 1 serving

Ingredients:

- 1 slice whole grain bread

- 1/2 ripe avocado

- 1 tsp sesame seeds (for calcium)

- Salt and pepper to taste

Nutritional Content (per serving):

- Calories: 250 kcal

- Calcium: 5% DV

- Protein: 6g

- Fiber: 7g

Preparation Instructions:

1. Toast the whole grain bread slice.

2. Mash the avocado and spread it on the toast.

3. Sprinkle sesame seeds, salt, and pepper on top.

4. Serve immediately.

Health Benefit:

Avocado provides healthy fats, and the whole grain bread offers fiber. Sesame seeds add a calcium boost, making this a nutritious and satisfying snack.

37. Roasted Chickpeas

Prep Time: 5 minutes || Cook Time: 30 minutes ||
Serving Size: 2 servings

Ingredients:

- 1 can chickpeas, drained and rinsed

- 1 tbsp olive oil

- 1 tsp paprika

- Salt to taste

Nutritional Content (per serving):

- Calories: 180 kcal

- Protein: 6g

- Fiber: 6g

- Calcium: 5% DV

Preparation Instructions:

1. Preheat oven to 400°F (200°C).
2. Toss chickpeas with olive oil, paprika, and salt.
3. Spread on a baking sheet and roast for 30 minutes, stirring occasionally, until crispy.
4. Serve warm or at room temperature.

Health Benefit:

Chickpeas are a great source of protein and fiber, essential for maintaining bone health. This snack is a healthy, crunchy alternative to traditional fried snacks.

38. Apple Slices with Almond Butter

Prep Time: 5 minutes || Serving Size: 1 serving

Ingredients:

- 1 apple, sliced

- 2 tbsp almond butter (rich in calcium and healthy fats)

Nutritional Content (per serving):

- Calories: 280 kcal

- Calcium: 8% DV

- Protein: 6g

- Fiber: 4g

Preparation Instructions:

1. Slice the apple.

2. Serve with almond butter for dipping.

Health Benefit:

Apples provide fiber and vitamins, while almond butter offers a good source of calcium and healthy fats, making this a simple yet beneficial snack for bone health.

39. Carrot and Raisin Salad

Prep Time: 10 minutes || Serving Size: 2 servings

Ingredients:

- 2 carrots, grated

- 1/4 cup raisins

- 2 tbsp Greek yogurt

- 1 tsp honey

- 1 tsp lemon juice

***Nutritional Content (per serving):**

- Calories: 120 kcal

- Calcium: 5% DV

- Protein: 2g

- Fiber: 3g

***Preparation Instructions:**

1. In a bowl, mix grated carrots and raisins.
2. In a separate bowl, whisk together Greek yogurt, honey, and lemon juice.
3. Pour dressing over the carrot mixture and toss well.
4. Serve chilled.

***Health Benefit:**

Carrots are high in vitamins and fiber. Greek yogurt adds a calcium boost, and raisins provide natural sweetness, making this salad a healthy, refreshing snack.

Prep Time: 5 minutes || Cook Time: 5 minutes

Serving Size: 2 servings

Ingredients:

- 1 cup edamame, shelled

- 1 tsp sea salt

Nutritional Content (per serving):

- Calories: 100 kcal

- Protein: 8g

- Fiber: 4g

- Calcium: 5% DV

Preparation Instructions:

1. Boil edamame in salted water for 5 minutes, then drain.

2. Sprinkle with sea salt.

3. Serve warm or at room temperature.

Health Benefit:

Edamame is a great source of protein and fiber. It's a simple, nutritious snack that's beneficial for maintaining healthy bones.

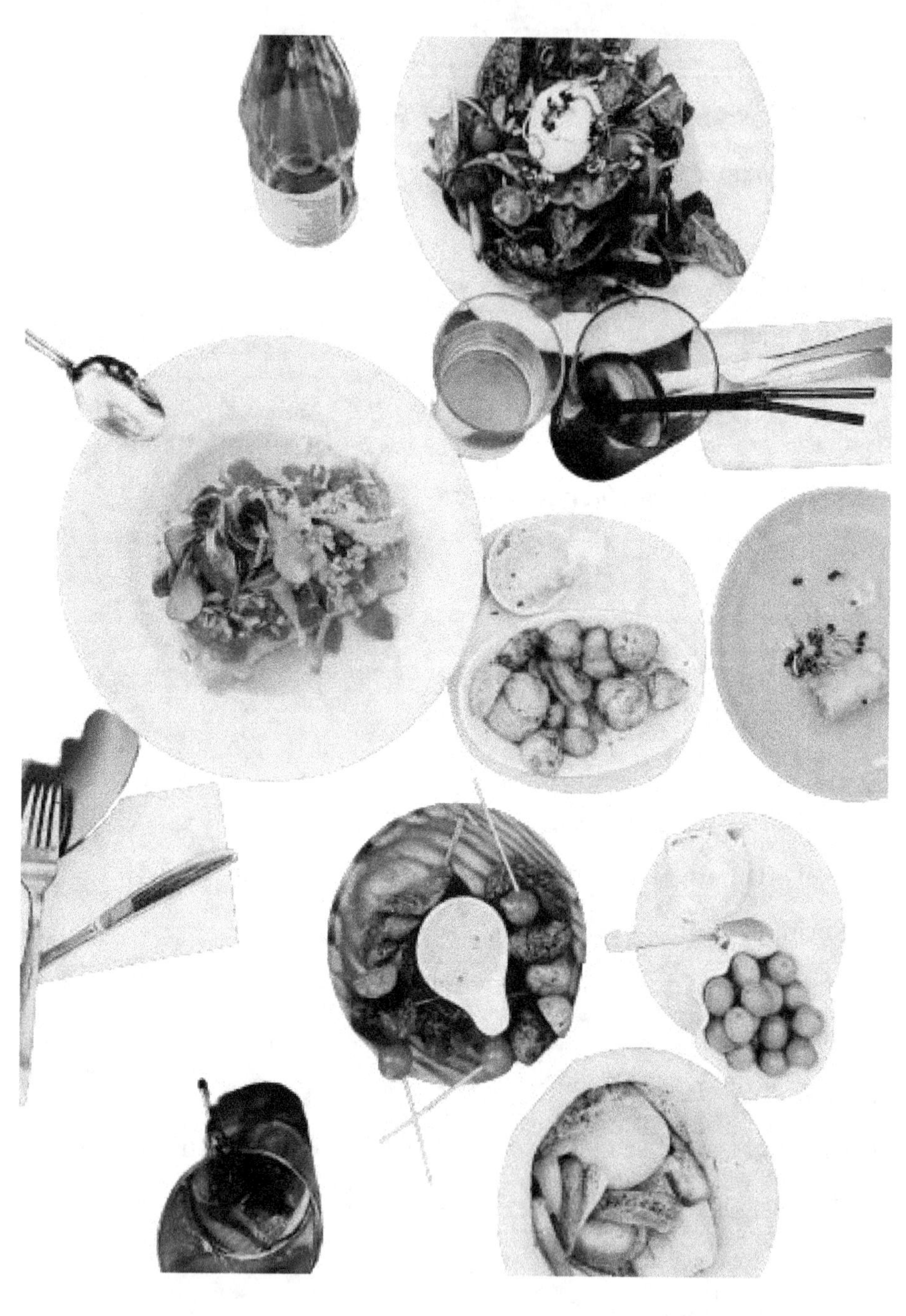

7. DESSERTS AND SWEET TREATS

41. Baked Apple with Walnuts and Honey

Prep Time: 5 minutes || Cook Time: 30 minutes ||
Serving Size: 2 servings

Ingredients:

- 2 apples, cored

- 1/4 cup walnuts, chopped (rich in omega-3 fatty acids)

- 2 tbsp honey

- 1/2 tsp cinnamon

Nutritional Content (per serving):

- Calories: 210 kcal

- Calcium: 2% DV

- Fiber: 5g

- Protein: 2g

Preparation Instructions:

1. Preheat oven to 350°F (175°C).

2. Place apples in a baking dish. Fill each apple's core with walnuts.

3. Drizzle honey and sprinkle cinnamon over apples.

4. Bake for 30 minutes, or until apples are tender.

5. Serve warm.

Health Benefit:

Apples and walnuts provide a healthy dose of antioxidants and omega-3 fatty acids, beneficial for bone health. This dessert is a naturally sweet treat without added sugars.

42. Greek Yogurt and Berry Freeze

***Prep Time: 5 minutes || Freezing Time: 2 hours ||
Serving Size: 4 servings***

Ingredients:

- 2 cups Greek yogurt (rich in calcium and protein)

- 1/2 cup mixed berries

- 2 tbsp honey

Nutritional Content (per serving):

- Calories: 150 kcal

- Calcium: 15% DV

- Protein: 10g

- Fiber: 1g

Preparation Instructions:

1. Mix Greek yogurt, berries, and honey in a bowl.

2. Spread the mixture in a shallow pan.

3. Freeze for 2 hours, or until set.

4. Break into pieces and serve.

Health Benefit:

Greek yogurt provides a good source of calcium and protein, essential for bone health. Berries add antioxidants and natural sweetness to this refreshing frozen dessert.

43. Dark Chocolate and Almond Bark

Prep Time: 10 minutes || Cook Time: 5 minutes (melting chocolate) || Chilling Time: 30 minutes || Serving Size: 6 servings

Ingredients:

- 100g dark chocolate (at least 70% cocoa)

- 1/4 cup almonds, chopped (for calcium and healthy fats)

- 1/4 cup dried cranberries

Nutritional Content (per serving):

- Calories: 150 kcal

- Calcium: 4% DV

- Fiber: 2g

- Protein: 3g

Preparation Instructions:

1. Melt dark chocolate in a heatproof bowl over a pot of simmering water.
2. Stir in chopped almonds and dried cranberries.
3. Spread the mixture on a baking sheet lined with parchment paper.
4. Chill in the refrigerator for 30 minutes, or until set.
5. Break into pieces and serve.

Health Benefit:

Dark chocolate is rich in antioxidants. Almonds add a healthy source of calcium and fats, making this a bone-friendly sweet treat in moderation.

Prep Time: 5 minutes || Chill Time: 2 hours ||
Serving Size: 2 servings

Ingredients:

- 1/4 cup chia seeds (rich in omega-3s)

- 1 cup almond milk, fortified

- 1 tbsp maple syrup

- 1/2 tsp vanilla extract

Nutritional Content (per serving):

- Calories: 200 kcal

- Calcium: 25% DV

- Fiber: 10g

- Protein: 5g

Preparation Instructions:

1. Mix chia seeds, almond milk, maple syrup, and vanilla extract in a bowl.

2. Refrigerate for at least 2 hours, or until the pudding achieves a thick consistency.

3. Stir before serving. Add more almond milk if needed.

Health Benefit:

Chia seeds are a great source of omega-3 fatty acids and fiber, essential for bone health. Fortified almond milk adds additional calcium to this simple, nutritious dessert.

45. Fruit Salad with Citrus Mint Dressing

Prep Time: 10 minutes || Serving Size: 4 servings

Ingredients:
- 1 cup strawberries, sliced
- 1 cup blueberries
- 1 orange, segmented
- 1 kiwi, sliced
- 1 tbsp fresh mint, chopped
- 2 tbsp orange juice
- 1 tsp honey

Nutritional Content (per serving):
- Calories: 80 kcal
- Calcium: 3% DV
- Fiber: 3g
- Protein: 1g

Preparation Instructions:

1. Combine strawberries, blueberries, orange segments, and kiwi in a large bowl.
2. In a small bowl, whisk together orange juice, honey, and chopped mint.
3. Pour the dressing over the fruit salad and toss gently.
4. Serve immediately or chill before serving.

Health Benefit:

This fruit salad is rich in vitamins and antioxidants, supporting overall health and bone strength. The citrus mint dressing adds a refreshing flavor without added sugars.

46. Oatmeal and Raisin Cookies

Prep Time: 10 minutes || Cook Time: 15 minutes ||
Serving Size: 12 cookies

Ingredients:

- 1 cup rolled oats
- 1/2 cup whole wheat flour
- 1/4 cup raisins
- 1/4 cup unsweetened applesauce
- 1/4 cup honey

- 1 egg

- 1/2 tsp cinnamon

- 1/4 tsp baking soda

Nutritional Content (per cookie):

- Calories: 90 kcal

- Calcium: 2% DV

- Fiber: 1g

- Protein: 2g

Preparation Instructions:

1. Preheat oven to 350°F (175°C).

2. Mix oats, flour, cinnamon, and baking soda in a bowl.

3. In another bowl, beat the egg with applesauce and honey.

4. Combine wet and dry ingredients, then fold in raisins.

5. Drop spoonfuls of the dough onto a baking sheet.

6. Bake for 15 minutes, or until golden.

7. Cool on a wire rack before serving.

Health Benefit:

Oats are high in fiber and low in fat, making these cookies a healthier alternative to traditional sugary desserts. The addition of whole wheat flour adds nutrients beneficial for bone health.

47. Carrot Cake with Cream Cheese Frosting

Prep Time: 20 minutes || Cook Time: 30 minutes || Serving Size: 8 servings

Ingredients:

- 2 cups grated carrots

- 1 1/2 cups whole wheat flour

- 1/2 cup unsweetened applesauce

- 1/2 cup honey

- 2 eggs

- 1 tsp baking soda

- 1 tsp cinnamon

- 1/2 cup low-fat cream cheese (for frosting)

- 2 tbsp honey (for frosting)

Nutritional Content (per serving):

- Calories: 220 kcal

- Calcium: 5% DV

- Fiber: 3g

- Protein: 5g

Preparation Instructions:

1. Preheat oven to 350°F (175°C).

2. Mix flour, baking soda, and cinnamon in a bowl.

3. In another bowl, beat eggs with applesauce and honey.

4. Combine wet and dry ingredients, then fold in grated carrots.

5. Pour batter into a greased baking pan and bake for 30 minutes.

6. For frosting, mix cream cheese with honey until smooth.

7. Once the cake is cooled, spread the frosting on top.

8. Serve and enjoy.

Health Benefit:

Carrot cake is a tasty way to consume vegetables. The whole wheat flour and carrots provide fiber, while the low-fat cream cheese frosting adds a touch of calcium.

48. Berry and Yogurt Smoothie

Prep Time: 5 minutes || Serving Size: 2 servings

Ingredients:

- 1 cup Greek yogurt (rich in calcium and protein)

- 1/2 cup mixed berries (for antioxidants)

- 1 banana

- 1/2 cup almond milk, fortified

- 1 tbsp honey

Nutritional Content (per serving):

- Calories: 180 kcal

- Calcium: 20% DV

- Protein: 10g

- Fiber: 3g

Preparation Instructions:

1. Place all ingredients in a blender.

2. Blend until smooth.

3. Serve immediately.

Health Benefit:

This smoothie combines the calcium and protein benefits of Greek yogurt with the vitamins and antioxidants of berries, making it a healthy and delicious dessert or snack.

49. Baked Pears with Cinnamon and Almonds

Prep Time: 5 minutes || Cook Time: 25 minutes || Serving Size: 2 servings

Ingredients:

- 2 pears, halved and cored

- 1/4 cup almonds, sliced (rich in calcium and healthy fats)

- 1/2 tsp cinnamon

- 2 tbsp honey

Nutritional Content (per serving):

- Calories: 200 kcal

- Calcium: 5% DV

- Fiber: 6g

- Protein: 3g

Preparation Instructions:

1. Preheat oven to 350°F (175°C).

2. Place pear halves face up in a baking dish.

3. Sprinkle each half with cinnamon and sliced almonds.

4. Drizzle honey over the pears.

5. Bake for 25 minutes, or until pears are tender.

6. Serve warm, possibly with a dollop of Greek yogurt.

Health Benefit:

Pears are a good source of fiber, and almonds provide healthy fats and calcium. The cinnamon adds flavor without extra sugar, making this a healthy and satisfying dessert for osteoporosis management.

50. Almond Flour Lemon Bars

Prep Time: 15 minutes || Cook Time: 25 minutes || Serving Size: 9 bars

Ingredients:

- 2 cups almond flour (rich in calcium)

- 1/2 cup coconut oil, melted

- 1/4 cup honey

- 2 lemons, juiced and zested

- 3 eggs

- 1 tsp vanilla extract

- Pinch of salt

Nutritional Content (per bar):

- Calories: 220 kcal

- Calcium: 6% DV

- Protein: 6g

- Fiber: 3g

Preparation Instructions:

1. Preheat oven to 350°F (175°C). Line a square baking dish with parchment paper.

2. Mix almond flour, salt, and melted coconut oil until crumbly. Press into the bottom of the baking dish.

3. Bake the crust for 10 minutes.

4. Whisk together eggs, honey, lemon juice, lemon zest, and vanilla extract.

5. Pour the lemon mixture over the baked crust.

6. Bake for an additional 15 minutes, or until the filling is set.

7. Cool in the pan, then chill in the fridge before cutting into bars.

Health Benefit:

Almond flour provides a gluten-free, high-calcium base, beneficial for bone health. The lemon adds vitamin C, essential for collagen production, making these bars a refreshing and healthier dessert option.

51. Bone-Building Green Smoothie

Prep Time: 5 minutes || Serving Size: 1 serving

Ingredients:

- 1 cup spinach (rich in calcium and vitamin K)

- 1/2 banana

- 1/2 cup fortified almond milk

- 1/2 cup Greek yogurt (rich in protein and calcium)

- 1 tbsp almond butter (for healthy fats and calcium)

- 1 tsp honey (optional)

Nutritional Content (per serving):

- Calories: 250 kcal

- Calcium: 30% DV

- Protein: 15g

- Fiber: 3g

Preparation Instructions:

1. Place all ingredients in a blender.

2. Blend until smooth and creamy.

3. Serve immediately.

Health Benefit:

This smoothie is packed with calcium and vitamin K from spinach, protein from Greek yogurt, and healthy fats from almond butter, making it an ideal beverage for bone health.

52. Turmeric Golden Milk

Prep Time: 5 minutes || Cook Time: 10 minutes || Serving Size: 1 serving

Ingredients:

- 1 cup fortified almond milk

- 1/2 tsp turmeric powder

- 1/4 tsp ginger powder

- 1/4 tsp cinnamon

- 1 tsp honey

- A pinch of black pepper

Nutritional Content (per serving):

- Calories: 60 kcal

- Calcium: 20% DV

- Protein: 1g

- Fiber: 0g

Preparation Instructions:

1. Heat almond milk in a pot over medium heat.

2. Add turmeric, ginger, cinnamon, black pepper, and honey.

3. Whisk continuously until warm and well-mixed.

4. Serve hot.

Health Benefit:

Turmeric and ginger are known for their anti-inflammatory properties, which can be beneficial for bone health. Fortified almond milk adds a good source of calcium.

53. Herbal Bone Strengthening Tea

Prep Time: 5 minutes || Cook Time: 10 minutes ||
Serving Size: 1 serving

Ingredients:

- 1 cup water

- 1 tsp dried nettle leaves (rich in calcium)

- 1 tsp dried horsetail (silica for bone health)

- Honey to taste

Nutritional Content (per serving):

- Calories: 0 kcal (without honey)

- Calcium: 5% DV

- Protein: 0g

- Fiber: 0g

Preparation Instructions:

1. Boil water and pour over nettle and horsetail leaves in a cup.

2. Steep for 10 minutes.

3. Strain and add honey to taste.

4. Serve warm.

Health Benefit:

Nettle leaves and horsetail are herbal remedies traditionally used for bone health due to their high mineral content, especially silica and calcium.

Prep Time: 5 minutes || Serving Size: 1 serving

Ingredients:

- 1/2 cup blueberries (for antioxidants)

- 1 cup spinach (rich in calcium and vitamin K)

- 1 banana

- 1/2 cup Greek yogurt (rich in protein and calcium)

- 1/2 cup orange juice (for vitamin C)

Nutritional Content (per serving):

- Calories: 220 kcal

- Calcium: 20% DV

- Protein: 10g

- Fiber: 4g

Preparation Instructions:

1. Place all ingredients in a blender.

2. Blend until smooth.

3. Serve immediately.

Health Benefit:

This smoothie is a powerhouse of bone-strengthening nutrients, including calcium from spinach and Greek yogurt, vitamin C from orange juice, and antioxidants from blueberries.

55. Calcium-Fortified Orange Juice

Serving Size: 1 serving

Ingredients:

- 1 cup fortified orange juice (rich in calcium and vitamin C)

Nutritional Content (per serving):

- Calories: 120 kcal
- Calcium: 30% DV
- Vitamin C: 100% DV
- Protein: 2g

Preparation Instructions:

1. Simply pour a cup of fortified orange juice into a glass.
2. Serve chilled.

Health Benefit:

Fortified orange juice is an easy and delicious way to consume extra calcium and vitamin C, which are essential for bone health.

Prep Time: 5 minutes || Cook Time: 5 minutes ||
Serving Size: 1 serving

Ingredients:

- 1 tsp matcha green tea powder

- 1 cup fortified almond milk

- 1 tsp honey (optional)

Nutritional Content (per serving):

- Calories: 70 kcal

- Calcium: 20% DV

- Protein: 1g

- Fiber: 1g

Preparation Instructions:

1. Heat almond milk in a pot, but do not boil.

2. Whisk in matcha powder until smooth.

3. Sweeten with honey if desired.

4. Serve warm.

Health Benefit:

Matcha is high in antioxidants, and fortified almond milk provides a good source of calcium. This latte is a bone-healthy alternative to coffee.

Prep Time: 5 minutes || Cook Time: 5 minutes ||
Serving Size: 1 serving

Ingredients:

- 1 cup fortified almond milk

- 2 tbsp unsweetened cocoa powder

- 1 tbsp honey or maple syrup

- A pinch of cinnamon

Nutritional Content (per serving):

- Calories: 100 kcal

- Calcium: 20% DV

- Protein: 2g

- Fiber: 2g

Preparation Instructions:

1. Heat almond milk in a pot over medium heat.

2. Add cocoa powder, honey or maple syrup, and cinnamon.

3. Whisk until well combined and warm.

4. Serve hot.

Health Benefit:

Cocoa is rich in flavonoids, which are good for heart health and may benefit bones. The fortified almond milk increases the calcium content, essential for bone strength.

58. Lemon Ginger Detox Drink

Prep Time: 5 minutes || Serving Size: 1 serving

Ingredients:

- 1 cup water

- 1/2 lemon, juiced

- 1/2 tsp grated ginger

- 1 tsp honey (optional)

Nutritional Content (per serving):

- Calories: 10 kcal (without honey)

- Calcium: 1% DV

- Vitamin C: 25% DV

- Protein: 0g

Preparation Instructions:

1. Mix lemon juice, grated ginger, and honey in a glass of water.

2. Stir well.

3. Serve at room temperature or chilled.

Health Benefit:

Lemon and ginger both have anti-inflammatory properties. Lemon provides vitamin C, essential for collagen formation, supporting bone health.

59. Pomegranate and Beet Juice

Prep Time: 10 minutes || Serving Size: 1 serving

Ingredients:

- 1/2 cup pomegranate juice (rich in antioxidants)

- 1/2 cup beet juice (for nitrates and minerals)

- 1/2 cup water

- 1 tsp lemon juice

Nutritional Content (per serving):

- Calories: 80 kcal

- Calcium: 2% DV

- Vitamin C: 15% DV

- Protein: 1g

Preparation Instructions:

1. Combine pomegranate juice, beet juice, water, and lemon juice in a glass.
2. Stir well.
3. Serve chilled.

Health Benefit:

Pomegranate and beet juices are both high in antioxidants and nutrients that support cardiovascular health, which is important for overall well-being including bone health.

60. Cucumber and Mint Infused Water

**Prep Time: 5 minutes || Chilling Time: 1 hour ||
Serving Size: 1 serving**

Ingredients:

- 1 cup water
- 1/2 cucumber, sliced
- 5-6 mint leaves

Nutritional Content (per serving):

- Calories: 0 kcal
- Calcium: 1% DV

- Protein: 0g

- Fiber: 0g

Preparation Instructions:

1. Place cucumber slices and mint leaves in a glass.

2. Fill the glass with water.

3. Refrigerate for at least 1 hour to infuse the flavors.

4. Serve chilled.

Health Benefit:

Cucumber and mint infused water is a refreshing and hydrating drink, important for maintaining overall health and supporting the body's natural bone maintenance processes.

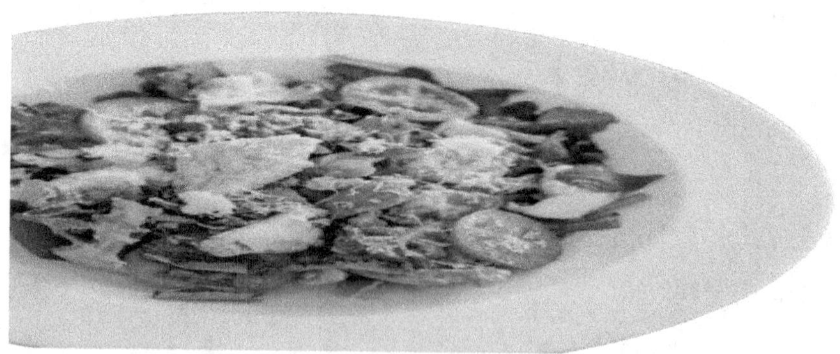

9. 14-DAY FLEXIBLE MEAL PLAN FOR OSTEOPOROSIS MANAGEMENT

WEEK 1: DAY 1 TO DAY 7

Day 1:

- Breakfast: Fortified Oatmeal Variations (#1)
- Lunch: Hearty Salmon Salad (#11)
- Dinner: Baked Lemon-Garlic Salmon (#21)
- Snacks: Greek Yogurt and Mixed Berry Parfait (#31), Carrot and Raisin Salad (#39)

Day 2:

- Breakfast: Protein-Packed Smoothies (#2)
- Lunch: Quinoa and Black Bean Bowl (#12)
- Dinner: Grilled Chicken and Vegetable Kabobs (#22)
- Snacks: Almond and Date Energy Balls (#32), Apple Slices with Almond Butter (#38)

Day 3:

- Breakfast: Calcium-Rich Pancakes and Waffles (#3)
- Lunch: Tofu and Vegetable Stir-Fry (#13)
- Dinner: Vegetarian Stuffed Acorn Squash (#23)
- Snacks: Baked Kale Chips (#33), Edamame with Sea Salt (#40)

Day 4:

- Breakfast: Avocado and Egg Toast (#4)
- Lunch: Chicken Caesar Salad Wrap (#14)
- Dinner: Tofu and Broccoli Stir-Fry (#24)
- Snacks: Hummus and Veggie Sticks (#34), Greek Yogurt and Berry Freeze (#42)

Day 5:

- Breakfast: Spinach and Feta Omelette (#5)
- Lunch: Mediterranean Chickpea Salad (#15)
- Dinner: Lentil and Vegetable Stew (#25)
- Snacks: Cottage Cheese with Pineapple (#35), Dark Chocolate and Almond Bark (#43)

Day 6:

- Breakfast: Quinoa Breakfast Bowl (#6)
- Lunch: Broccoli and Cheese Stuffed Baked Potato (#16)
- Dinner: Grilled Tofu with Lemon Herb Quinoa (#26)
- Snacks: Avocado Toast with Sesame Seeds (#36), Chia Seed Pudding (#44)

Day 7:

- Breakfast: Greek Yogurt with Mixed Berries (#7)

- Lunch: Lentil Soup with Spinach (#17)

- Dinner: Baked Cod with Tomato and Olive Tapenade (#27)

- Snacks: Roasted Chickpeas (#37), Fruit Salad with Citrus Mint Dressing (#45)

WEEK 2: DAY 8 TO DAY 14

Day 8:

- Breakfast: Almond Butter and Banana Smoothie (#8)

- Lunch: Turkey and Avocado Wrap (#18)

- Dinner: Spinach and Ricotta Stuffed Chicken Breast (#28)

- Snacks: Baked Apple with Walnuts and Honey (#41), Oatmeal and Raisin Cookies (#46)

Day 9:

- Breakfast: Kale and Mushroom Breakfast Saute (#9)

- Lunch: Sweet Potato and Black Bean Chili (#19)

- Dinner: Butternut Squash Risotto (#29)

- Snacks: Greek Yogurt and Mixed Berry Parfait (#31), Carrot Cake with Cream Cheese Frosting (#47)

Day 10:

- Breakfast: Cottage Cheese and Pineapple Bowl (#10)
- Lunch: Hearty Salmon Salad (#11)
- Dinner: Grilled Vegetable and Halloumi Skewers (#30)
- Snacks: Almond and Date Energy Balls (#32), Berry and Yogurt Smoothie (#48)

Day 11:

- Breakfast: Protein-Packed Smoothies (#2)
- Lunch: Quinoa and Black Bean Bowl (#12)
- Dinner: Baked Lemon-Garlic Salmon (#21)
- Snacks: Baked Kale Chips (#33), Baked Pears with Cinnamon and Almonds (#49)

Day 12:

- Breakfast: Calcium-Rich Pancakes and Waffles (#3)
- Lunch: Tofu and Vegetable Stir-Fry (#13)
- Dinner: Vegetarian Stuffed Acorn Squash (#23)
- Snacks: Hummus and Veggie Sticks (#34), Almond Flour Lemon Bars (#50)

Day 13:

- Breakfast: Avocado and Egg Toast (#4)
- Lunch: Chicken Caesar Salad Wrap (#14)
- Dinner: Tofu and Broccoli Stir-Fry (#24)
- Snacks: Cottage Cheese with Pineapple (#35), Greek Yogurt and Berry Freeze (#42)

Day 14:

- Breakfast: Spinach and Feta Omelette (#5)
- Lunch: Mediterranean Chickpea Salad (#15)
- Dinner: Lentil and Vegetable Stew (#25)
- Snacks: Avocado Toast with Sesame Seeds (#36), Fruit Salad with Citrus Mint Dressing (#45)

This 14-Day Flexible Meal Plan has been expertly crafted to offer a diverse and well-rounded diet that promotes strong bones and overall health. Feel free to swap out recipes to suit your personal tastes and dietary requirements, making sure that each day is both nourishing and pleasurable.

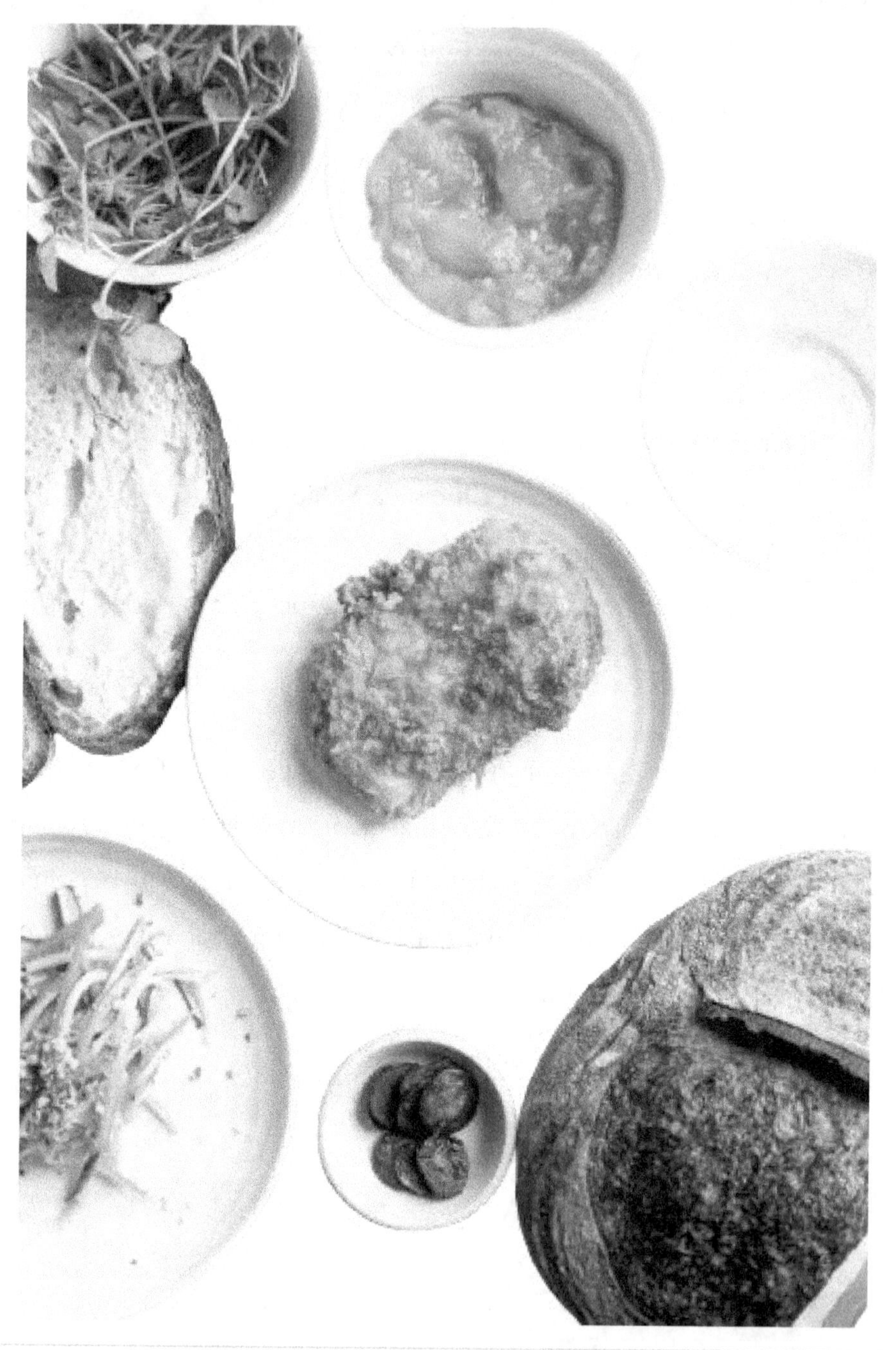

10. SPECIAL SECTION: ADVANCED COOKING TECHNIqUES AND HOLISTIC TIPS

In this section, we explore the intricacies of cooking and meal preparation, with a special emphasis on enhancing bone health. This is particularly beneficial for individuals who are dealing with osteoporosis. It offers in-depth knowledge, practical illustrations, and helpful suggestions to present a comprehensive guide.

ADVANCED COOKING METHODS FOR NUTRIENT PRESERVATION

1. ***Sous-Vide Cooking:*** This method entails cooking food in a sealed bag submerged in a water bath at precise temperatures. It's great for preserving the nutritional value and enhancing the taste of proteins, without the need for extra fats. This makes it perfect for lean meats and omega-3 rich fish.

2. ***Roasting with Herbs:*** Enhance the flavor and nutritional value of your vegetables and meats by roasting them with bone-health-promoting herbs. Thyme, known for its anti-inflammatory

properties, can support bone health while adding a delicious taste to your dishes.

3. ***Infusing Broths:*** Crafting your own broths using bones, vegetables, and herbs is a fantastic method for extracting essential minerals such as calcium and magnesium. Simmering bones slowly can release important nutrients like collagen, glucosamine, and calcium, which are crucial for maintaining strong bones.

TAILORED MEAL PREPPING STRATEGIES

1. ***Thematic Meal Planning:*** Incorporate weekly themes into your meal planning to add variety to your diet and ensure you're getting all the essential nutrients for bone health. For example, you can have "Mediterranean Mondays" or "Fish Fridays".

2. ***Snack Smart:*** Pair protein with a calcium source for optimal snacking. For example, you can enjoy almond butter on whole grain toast or pair cheese with apple slices. This combination not only fulfills your cravings but also offers a snack that is packed with essential nutrients.

3. ***Personalized Portioning:*** Freeze meals in individual servings, taking into account unique nutritional requirements and appetite. Each meal is carefully crafted to suit your specific dietary needs.

ENHANCED SHOPPING AND STORAGE TECHNIQUES

1. ***Exploring the Glycemic Index of Fruits and Vegetables:*** Opting for fruits and vegetables with a lower glycemic index, such as berries and leafy greens, can contribute to maintaining a healthy weight, which is important for minimizing strain on bones.

2. ***Making Ethical and Organic Choices:*** Whenever you can, choose organic produce to minimize your exposure to pesticides, which can have an impact on your bone health. Opting for ethical choices, such as grass-fed meats, can enhance the nutrient quality of your meals.

3. ***Creative Storage Solutions:*** Utilize vacuum-sealed containers to extend the shelf life of your food. Freezing herbs in olive oil is a great way to retain their nutrients and make them easily accessible for cooking purposes.

1. Superfoods: Incorporate nutrient-rich foods that promote bone health, such as salmon (packed with vitamin D and omega-3s), almonds (abundant in calcium and magnesium), and tofu (containing isoflavones that may support bone density).

2. Gut-Healthy Fermented Foods: Add kefir and sauerkraut to your diet for improved gut health. Having a healthy gut is crucial for better absorption of essential minerals like calcium, which is vital for maintaining strong bones.

3. Spices and Herbs: Incorporate turmeric, ginger, and black pepper into your dishes to enhance both taste and take advantage of their anti-inflammatory benefits. Studies have shown that long-term inflammation can contribute to a decrease in bone density.

EXPERT TIPS ON HYDRATION

1. Staying Hydrated for Stronger Bones: Hydration plays a vital role in maintaining bone health. Discover the wonderful world of herbal teas and infusions, which not only keep you hydrated but also offer a wealth of minerals and antioxidants.

2. Mineral Water: Choose mineral water as it contains trace minerals such as magnesium, which is essential for maintaining strong bones.

With the inclusion of these advanced cooking techniques, meal prepping strategies, and shopping tips, people can greatly improve the nutritional value of their diets. This all-encompassing approach to food and nutrition goes beyond just addressing osteoporosis; it encourages a lifestyle that promotes overall health and well-being.

This valuable resource combines cutting-edge research with practical cooking tips, providing a comprehensive guide for individuals seeking to enhance their bone health through mindful cooking and dietary choices.

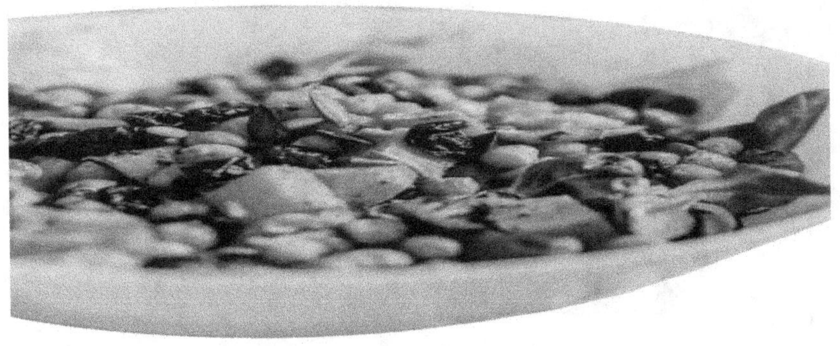

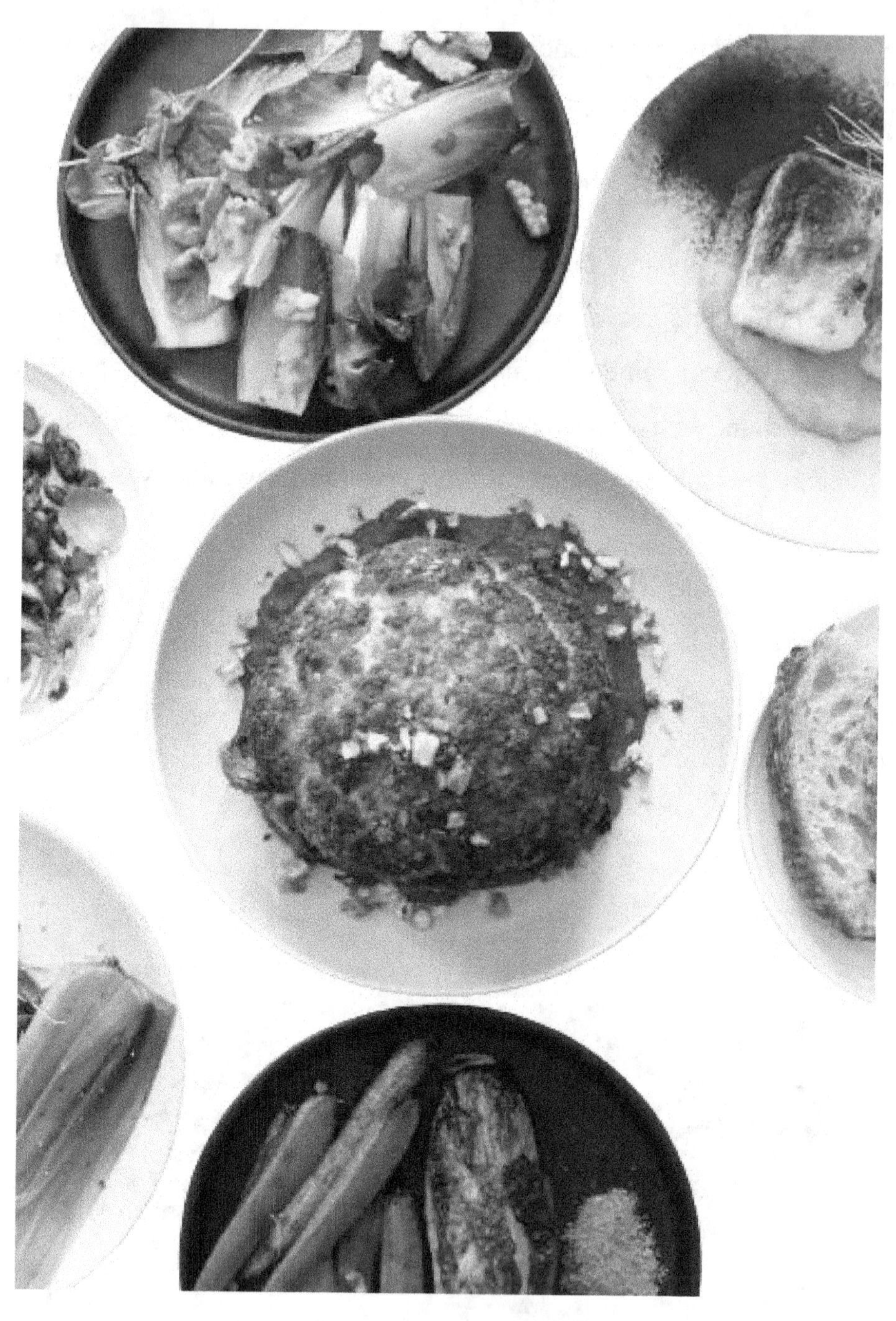

CONCLUSION

As we reach the end of the "Osteoporosis Cookbook," it's crucial to recognize that this book goes beyond just providing recipes. It serves as a helpful companion and a valuable resource for individuals navigating osteoporosis with the help of nutrition. Every recipe is designed to not only provide a delicious meal, but also contribute to your overall health and well-being.

We've prepared a 14-Day Flexible Meal Plan to help you along your culinary adventure. This plan offers a well-organized method for integrating the recipes from this cookbook into your everyday routine, guaranteeing a diverse and nutritious diet that promotes strong bones. The plan is flexible, giving you the freedom to combine recipes based on your personal tastes and requirements.

This meal plan is crafted to offer versatility and can be easily customized to suit personal preferences, dietary limitations, and nutritional requirements. This guide is designed to assist you in seamlessly integrating bone-healthy eating habits into your daily routine.

The "Osteoporosis Cookbook" aims to provide a wide range of tasty and nourishing recipes that promote strong bones and overall health. As you begin your culinary adventure, your feedback and experiences are highly valuable. Sharing a review or your personal story can not only provide us with valuable feedback but also inspire and encourage others in similar situations.

Keep in mind that dealing with osteoporosis requires a holistic approach, including making changes to your diet, engaging in regular exercise, and adopting a positive lifestyle. This cookbook is designed to be a trusted guide for those seeking to improve their well-being. It is packed with nutritious recipes and practical advice to help you achieve stronger bones and a healthier lifestyle.

HAPPY COOKING!